The New
Thriving
Medical Practice

How to Get Off the Hamster Wheel,
Work Smarter (Not Harder),
Generate More Revenue,
and Enjoy Greater Career Satisfaction
in a Post-Pandemic World

Patrick Phillips and Vicki Rackner, MD

Foreword by
Malik Handoush, CMRM

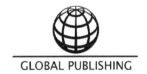

GLOBAL PUBLISHING

Global Publishing
Fort Worth, Texas

This publication is designed to provide accurate and authoritative information in regard to the subject matter covered. It is sold with the understanding that the authors and publisher are not engaged in rendering legal, accounting or other professional services or advice. If legal advice or other expert assistance is required, the services of a competent professional should be sought.

ISBN paperback print edition: 978-0-9966097-1-5
Printed in the United States of America

Library of Congress Cataloging-in-Publication Data
Phillips, Patrick
Rackner, Vicki

The New Thriving Medical Practice
How to Get Off the Hamster Wheel, Work Smarter (Not Harder), Generate More Revenue, and Enjoy Greater Career Satisfaction in a Post-Pandemic World

0522A

Table of Contents

FOREWORD

Every physician dreams of having a thriving medical practice. Even if they work for a hospital or large medical group, most doctors would prefer to be their own boss and run a profitable private practice. This book can show you how this can be possible for every physician or practice manager who puts the best practices described in this book to work in their own practice.

My colleagues, Patrick Phillips and Dr. Vicki Rackner, have cracked the code on private practice profitability. Their combined five decades of contact and observation in the medical field have given them insight and practical experience that can help any physician to thrive in their own private practice.

As a practicing, general surgeon, Dr. Rackner faced the challenges all doctors face: how to provide optimal medical services to patients while making sure the bills get paid (and generate enough profit so that the physician and their staff thrive in their personal lives as well.)

There are only so many hours in the day and so much time and energy that a doctor can devote to making sure her patients get optimal medical care. At the same time, she has an obligation to those working with her to make sure they are all compensated fairly and that there are funds available to grow and expand the practice.

It is a common myth that doctors are all rich; that doctors earn above average incomes and that they have an abundance of wealth available to them for investing, travel, education, entertainment and an abundant lifestyle.

This is true in many cases, but the fact is that physician personal incomes have dropped drastically in the last few years and many are struggling to remain in private practice. Some are being forced to go to work as an employee for a large hospital or some impersonal medical group. They, in effect, are simply putting in the time that others dictate and working for whatever someone else thinks they are worth.

This book can show you the light at the end of the tunnel. Whether you are a doctor fighting to keep your private practice open due to a lack of revenue (or perhaps mismanaging the expenses in your practice) or someone who works in management, you will find the suggestions in this book to be invaluable. Many struggling practices have been turned into profitable entities after putting these practical ideas into practice. You, too, can thrive in your own private practice.

As owner and manager of a local office of the nation's largest network of Certified Medical Revenue Managers, I am happy to be able to share this book with you. I am available anytime for consulting with you on how to implement new ways of cutting expenses and increasing your revenue.

Sincerely,

Malik Handoush, CMRM
Rising Sun Partners
Malik@Risingsunpartners.com
Risingsunpartners.com
(904) 526-8991

PREFACE

Would you like to build a thriving medical practice in this time of radical change? If so, then you have come to the right place.

You will benefit from two unique perspectives. Both of your co-authors have been in the medical trenches and understand the day-to-day challenges physicians like yourself face. Furthermore, they both have experience in helping their clients transform their practices.

Vicki Rackner MD is a surgeon by training. After running a solo private practice for many years, she launched her consulting company in 2000, helping physicians get better outcomes. She is the author of several books, a nationally recognized keynote speaker and a business coach for physicians nationwide.

Patrick Phillips, formerly with Apple Computer, is Chairman of the Medical Revenue Management Association of America and editorial board member of Billing and Coding Advantage Magazine. He has helped hundreds of physicians put more money in their pockets since 1994.

Our combined backgrounds in delivering clinical medicine and growing medical practices make us uniquely qualified to help you achieve the personal, professional and financial rewards that initially attracted you to a career in medicine.

Since we are both contributing to this book, it will probably be clear when we are relating something specifically personal about either of us. Otherwise, you can just sit back and enjoy our "mind meld" as we guide you to greater success in your practice.

THE FORMULA FOR MEDICAL PRACTICE SUCCESS

The formula for practice success was simple when Vicki began her medical career thirty years ago. Her mentor advised, **"Take good care of patients, and everything else will take care of itself."**

Today, taking good care of patients is necessary but no longer sufficient to build a successful practice.

Vicki believes that the promise of medicine can still be realized. However, the path has changed. This book is your roadmap.

WHY SHOULD YOU LISTEN TO US?

VICKI: Both as a physician running a private practice and an entrepreneur, I, like you, have asked, "How do I respond to changing times?"

Very briefly, here's my story. I decided to be a doctor as I woke from my own lifesaving operation at age 23. Not surprisingly I became a general surgeon.

I've run my own private practice, served as a faculty member at the University of Washington School of Medicine and had the honor of treating tens of thousands of patients.

In 1998 I took a leave from my practice to be a full-time family caregiver. I generated income as an expert reviewing medical malpractice lawsuits.

When a turbulent caregiving year came to an end, it was time to step back into full-time work. In 2000, I launched my consulting practice helping doctors, patients and family caregivers partner more effectively.

You might imagine that building this business would be easy. After all, everyone wants better medical outcomes at a lower cost.

I spent many years struggling to grow my business, and I came to understand that I faced a systems challenge. As a physician I was wired differently than business-minded people.

If I wanted to succeed as a consultant and entrepreneur, I needed to understand how the world of business worked.

I read books about sales and marketing, attended seminars about creating and distributing intellectual property, and studied the best practices of thought leaders. I hired mentors who taught me the importance of seeing my value through my clients' eyes and positioning myself as an expert.

Once I cracked the business code, I saw a complete transformation in the results I got.

PATRICK: Since 1987 I have worked with hundreds of billing professionals and doctors from almost every known specialty to help them manage their revenue and build more profitable practices. Many of them were struggling to figure out how to make their practice profitable. I don't mean they were trying to get rich; many of them were just trying to stay in private practice and pay their bills.

However, all of them were desperately trying to understand, as Dr. Rackner says, how the world of business worked.

Because, as much as you might like to think that your medical practice is simply a provider of medical services, the reality is that your practice must make a profit at the end of each month in order to continue to provide those services.

Let me repeat that.

The reality is that your practice must make a profit at the end of each month in order to continue to provide medical services.

And if your personal income is not providing you and your family with what you need to live a happy, satisfied life, you will become negative, miserable and discouraged. You must agree that this would help no one.

Stay with us. There is hope. There is a way for you to do what you love and make the money you need to provide you and your family with the lifestyle you deserve.

WHAT DOES THIS HAVE TO DO WITH YOU?

Historically, physicians could be very successful without paying much attention to the business side of medicine.

This is no longer true.

You see how the Affordable Care Act is impacting your practice. You may be experiencing:

- Shifting referral patterns as physicians sell their practices
- Concerns about cash flow with ICD-10
- Rising costs
- Falling fees
- New compliance issues, like the use of EMR's

You cannot fix these problems by seeing more patients. The status quo - the way you've always done things - offers limited utility in addressing these issues. Successful physicians must see their practices differently.

THE POST-OBAMACARE ERA PRESENTS BUSINESS CHALLENGES

The truth is that today you face classic business challenges:

- How do you attract and retain patients?
- How do you hold down costs?
- How do you increase your revenue by working smarter and not harder?

You need business savvy to answer these questions.

You can transform your practice and accelerate your growth by learning more about how the world of business operates.

MONEY, MARKETING AND OTHER TABOO TOPICS

The biggest barrier to your practice's growth may be a set of beliefs about what constitutes conduct becoming to a physician.

Our healthcare system is constructed around a core principle: you have a duty to deliver medical care regardless of a patient's ability to pay. But with this caring attitude towards helping patients, most physicians have learned to avoid conversations - or even thinking - about money.

It's time to rethink your relationship to money and marketing and other taboo topics. **You cannot serve patients if you cannot meet your payroll.**

You don't have to choose between running a profitable practice or dedicating yourself to service. You can have both.

Reinvention is the operative word.

Reinvention will help you achieve practice success in these rapidly changing times. You can reinvent the way you generate patient referrals. You can shed old marketing beliefs that weigh you down and adopt new practices that work in today's healthcare environment.

How can you transform your practice results?

Here are the steps that lead to sustained, measurable improvements for the physicians that Dr. Rackner coaches:

- Identify the activities that bring you true career satisfaction.
- Paint a picture of success and determine the income goals to support this vision.
- Explore what you value and what brings meaning to your life.
- Ask critical questions and challenge self-limiting thoughts.
- See the world through the eyes of patients and colleagues.
- Distinguish between what patients need and what they want.
- Take action.
- Acquire new skills and develop new habits.
- Assemble teams so you can stay in your wheelhouse.
- Measure outcomes and make course corrections.

At the end of each chapter, you will find action steps. While these steps are simple, they are not always easy to implement. Change can be difficult.

To make it easier, you will find new self-talk for physicians in Appendix A that replace self-limiting beliefs. Why is this so important? Consider these wise words:

"Watch your thoughts, they become words;

watch your words, they become actions;

watch your actions, they become habits;

watch your habits, they become character;

watch your character, for it becomes your destiny."

PRACTICE-BUILDING IS RELATIONSHIP-BUILDING

Some things never change. Practice-building has always been and will always be about relationship-building.

However, the way you connect with patients - and people who make referrals - is different today than it was 30 years ago.

Stay with us. We will show you how you can build your practice with strategies that:

- Maintain the highest level of professionalism.

- Make the most of your marketing resources.

- Produce results.

Grab a highlighter and let's get started.

INTRODUCTION

Even though Beth is an excellent orthopedic surgeon whom patients love, she is concerned about the future of her practice.

Her referrals are down 30% from last year, primarily because many of her referring physicians who sold their practices to the local hospital were required to refer patients internally.

Furthermore, she sees her professional fees going down and costs going up. One month she wondered whether she would have to tap into her 401K to meet her payroll. She recently met with a banker to take out a line of credit.

In her darker moments she wonders if she should seriously consider the hospital's offer to buy her practice. For her, though, that would mean selling out. She would rather just quit.

Her stress exacerbated her TMJ pain, and she knew she could no longer put off the dreaded dental work she tried so hard to avoid.

She made an appointment with her dentist who had treated her for 21 years. His secretary made a quotation error that was thousands of dollars off. He wouldn't stand behind it, so Beth decided it was time to leave his practice.

As she pondered where she would go, an email appeared in her in box saying, "Find a dentist near you." She clicked on the link and the dental office offered to call her. She replied to the email and included her phone number. The office called her in less than 60 seconds.

A few days later when she walked into the office that looked like a dental version of the Taj Mahal, she feared that her own dentist's revised quote might be half of what the new dentist would charge.

As she surveyed the waiting room, her eyes were drawn to the four receptionists, plasma TVs, laptops for patients' use and a self-service area with tea and coffee. All staff members were dressed in uniforms monogrammed with the company's logo.

Beth was promptly ushered into a treatment room where all the equipment was buried in wooden cabinets. She was offered a warm aromatherapy neck wrap and an iPod.

When the tech announced she wanted to take x-rays, Beth mentioned that she gagged easily. The tech said, "No problem; we'll take a full-mouth tomogram."

The dentist came in and conducted the exam. She dictated her assessment of every tooth in Beth's mouth to her assistant.

Then, the dentist outlined Beth's options in an unhurried way.

The quote for the work included a careful tooth-by-tooth assessment of what needed to be done and the cost for each element.

The practice offered a program for patients without dental insurance. Patients pay $180 a year and get two free cleanings, unlimited x-rays and exams, and 30% off all serious work.

Their quote ended up being half of her original dentist's.

Beth spent many hours in the dental chair. She was reminded by the staff, "Any time you want a break it's fine. Just let us know."

When Beth reported that her jaw was locking, the dentist put down the drill and massaged her masseter and temporalis muscles.

Beth considered how much she appreciated the attentive care she received.

There was something more. Suddenly she had a glimmer of hope.

What if she implemented only one or two of the innovative patient-centered ideas from her dental experience? She knew she could transform her practice.

You are responding to a radically changing health care environment. You also have access to technologies and interventions that can transform the way in which you attract patients to your practice and deliver patient care.

Paradoxically, the same forces that you may perceive as the problem, like your patients' online evaluation of your practice, can be part of your solution.

What Is the Reinvented Medical Practice?

Do you run a small business? Most physicians say, "No. I run a medical practice."

Thriving physicians KNOW they are running small businesses. Yes, it's a specialized hybrid business venture, but the process of building a successful business transcends the details of who is selling what to whom.

Yes, you are running a business too!

This idea may make you feel uncomfortable. It SHOULD make you feel uncomfortable. You have the training to care for patients; however, no one laid out the rules and tools to manage the business side of medicine.

- You learned how to take good care of patients. Who taught you how to attract and retain those patients?

- You learned how to interpret the I's & O's of an ICU patient. Who taught you how to interpret how cash flows in and out of your practice?

- You learned how to integrate technological advances into patient care. Who taught you how to leverage Facebook, blogs and YouTube to grow your practice?

Hockey great Wayne Gretzky said, "I skate to where the puck is going to be; not where it has been." Many forces are changing the trajectory of the "medical success puck."

The Post-Obamacare Era is your wake-up call telling you that it's time to switch strategies. Whether it continues unscathed, self-implodes or is repealed and replaced, the government will almost surely be involved in healthcare more and more. The physicians who ignore the business side of their practices do so at their own peril.

We're here to help you acquire the rules and tools you will need to join doctors who are thriving in the Post-Obamacare Era.

For many physicians this means leaving their comfort zones and learning new skills.

TRADITIONAL MEDICAL PRACTICES VS SMALL BUSINESSES

Let's compare and contrast the conventional medical practice and a conventional small business.

Here are some qualities you share with small business owners:

- You both generate revenue.
- You both manage employees.
- You both have expenses.
- You both pay taxes.
- You both use the revenue you generate to provide for your families.

The metrics by which you measure success separate you from a small business owner.

- **Small businesses** win by optimizing profits.
- It's fundamentally about financial outcomes.
- **Medical practices** win by optimizing the quality of medical care.
- It's fundamentally about clinical outcomes.
- However, these different paths lead to the same destination: generating revenue by delivering products or services or a transformation that people value.
- Patients are willing to exchange money for that value.

The formal training and skills that support success are different.

- Small business owners generally have training in sales, marketing and finance.

- You have formal training to perform diagnostic and therapeutic interventions.

- However, the most successful physicians and business owners master both sets of skills.

The relationship with the "stakeholders" - the people with a vested interest in the organization - is different.

- In small businesses, the consumer/customer/client generally makes purchasing choices, uses the product or service and pays the bill. Think about purchasing a car, booking a vacation or hiring someone to do yard work.

- In your practice, you manage complex triangulated relationships between yourself, the person who benefits from your care (the patient), the people and organizations that pay for the care, and the organizations that impose compliance standards. Each party wants different and often conflicting things.

- However, both physicians and small business owners succeed by identifying a buyer who is willing to exchange money for the value they deliver.

WHY SHOULD BUSINESS STRATEGIES MATTER TO YOU?

Today, patients are behaving more like consumers.

- **Patients are driving more healthcare choices.** They have access to medical information. They can initiate diagnostic and therapeutic interventions without physicians. They have more financial skin in the game, and there is greater transparency regarding pricing.

- **Patients increasingly drive referrals, either directly or indirectly.** They choose where and when they seek medical services in much the same way you book air travel: on the basis of cost and convenience and the overall experience.

> *When patients behave more like consumers, you optimize your chances of success by embracing sound business practices.*

What are the basic rules in the world of business?

Consumers exchange their money for the value they seek.

Value, like beauty, is in the eye of the beholder. Successful brands, from Apple to Nordstrom to Taylor Swift, regularly interact with their customers and fans to understand what's important to them.

Successful businesses understand that *what they think* is not nearly as important as *what their customers think*. When Steve Jobs left Apple, he set up a business called Next; he thought it would be the next Apple. The market disagreed.

When businesses want to increase prices, they deliver more value.

What do these rules mean for you?

You want to ask three questions:

1. Who is your customer?
2. What does your customer value?
3. Is the customer willing to exchange money for the products and services you offer?

Who is your customer? It depends:

- If you think of the customer as the person or organization who writes you a check, the insurance company is your functional buyer. Your patients who are responsible for ever-increasing co-pays and deductibles are also customers.

- If you think of the customer as the person or organization who makes purchasing choices, your referral sources are your customers. When patients arrive at your office, they have usually made a decision to get their medical care from you.

- If you think of the customer as the person who makes a transformation as a result of your medical care, the patient is your customer.

This is not an armchair academic exercise; this has real and practical applications. If you want to be successful, you must focus on the things that your customers value. Each stakeholder wants very different things.

- The insurance company rewards physicians who help them maximize profits. That's what they value.

- Referring physicians value quality care with optimal medical outcomes.

- Patients want something more than a medical outcome; they want an experience that helps them achieve a personal outcome.

In the post-Google era, patients increasingly drive referrals. They are your buyers. How well do you understand what your patients really want?

What if you ran your practice with the mindset that your patients are your true customers? That would mean that delivering care patients truly want - patient-centered care - is the key to success.

Think about that for a moment. Let this sink in:

Delivering care patients truly want - patient-centered care - is the key to success.

How Do Consumers Make Purchasing Choices?

Consumers behave irrationally. They make choices with their emotional brains and justify them with their thinking brains. Businesses have the greatest chance of success when they offer their buyer something that the buyer *really* wants.

Your patients behave irrationally, too. Poor medication compliance is a case in point. There is a reason patients do the things that they do, and once you understand what drives their behaviors, you are in a position to influence them.

Consumers have predictable barriers to making purchases.

Buyers' beliefs. The first time we were charged by an airline for carry-on luggage we were shocked; our belief is that carry-on luggage is free.

Some patients hold the beliefs that medical care should be free. A urologist asks, "How do I charge more when my patients have a heart attack in the waiting room when we ask for a $20 co-pay?"

You will certainly have patients that fall into this category; however, many patients will pay for the things that they value. At the height of the great recession, Americans paid billions of dollars out of pocket on weight loss, anti-aging therapies and nutritional supplements.

Your goal is to attract the patients who understand your value and are willing to pay for it. They are out there!

Buyers' priorities. Have you ever had patients who tell you they cannot afford medication, but find a way to smoke two packs of cigarettes a day? Generally, spending reflects underlying values.

Buyers' failure to see value. Businesses understand that it's their job to understand what customers want, and clearly lay out their value.

As a physician you value medical outcomes; patients value personal outcomes and the experience. They make choices about medical care in much the same way you make your air travel plans.

Buyers' failure to believe business claims. Sophisticated consumers have their guards up for fraud and hype. They simply may not believe the claims businesses make.

Have you ever seen TV commercials to promote the services of a bariatric surgeon? They generally do not feature the surgeon; they feature delighted patients with dramatic before-and-after pictures.

Buyers' forgetfulness. Your patients may know someone who needs your services, but forget about you in that moment.

Does this mean that you need marketing and sales skills?

The short answer is yes.

These are critical skills for any physician who wants to attract more patient referrals, motivate their staff to be kinder to grumpy patients and increase patient compliance.

Your ability to build rapport and influence others is a leadership skill that will serve you well at work, at home, and at play.

PHYSICIANS' OLD BELIEFS ABOUT SELLING

When Vicki entered medical school thirty years ago, she believed, "Doctors shouldn't sell; it's unprofessional."

Furthermore, she believed that she didn't have to sell. If she just took good care of patients, her practice would grow.

It was a different story when she traded her scalpel for a pen and a microphone and launched a career writing and speaking and consulting. She had to sell.

And almost every day as an entrepreneur she said to herself, "I hate selling!"

NEW BELIEFS ABOUT SALES AND MARKETING

Here's how Vicki made peace with sales and marketing.

She reframed marketing as the process of engaging someone in a conversation; she reframed selling as the process of inspiring someone to take action.

You sell every day. You sell when you persuade your kids to practice the piano, help a colleague see things your way or get your food prepared as you want it at a restaurant.

You sell when you persuade patients to take medication as prescribed, change lifestyle habits or follow up with a specialist.

How do physicians overcome the professional and ethical barriers to asking patients to pay them for the value they deliver?

Physicians have an ethical duty to provide medical care regardless of a patient's ability to pay. In other words, physicians should be blind to financial concerns. This sets up a culture in which physicians are taught not to talk about money with patients.

Patients want to talk about medical costs. They live with the economic realities of both illness and the cost of medical care. They expect to exchange money for the value they receive, just as they would with any other business transaction.

When you communicate the value you offer, it's easier for patients to understand and express a willingness to pay.

While it may feel uncomfortable to talk about money, you can learn how to do it with greater ease.

BEGIN WHERE YOU ARE AND TRANSFORM YOUR PRACTICE

Just as there is a system to evaluate and treat patients, so too is there a system for building a thriving practice that works for you. Here are the steps:

1. Identify your "sweet spot" where purpose, passion and profit meet.
2. Gather intelligence to clarify what your patients and referring physicians really want.
3. Put your best foot forward. You only have one chance to make a first impression.
4. Pave a path to your door. Create a culture of referrals.
5. Launch marketing campaigns that work.

Later we will explore your relationship to money, address how cash flows in and out of your practice, and examine how you build wealth.

Last, we will talk about how to offer leadership.

SUMMARY

- You are running a small business.
- The skills to run a successful practice are different than the skills that help you take care of patients.
- You can learn the rules and acquire the tools to run a thriving practice in the Post-Obamacare Era.

1

BECOMING REMARKABLE

When Vicki's son was in Little League, he wanted to buy an expensive bat. She asked the clerk why this bat cost so much more than the others. He said, "It has a big sweet spot."

Vicki asked, "What's a sweet spot?"

Her son answered, "That's the part of the bat that hits home runs."

You have a professional sweet spot. When your day-to-day activities fall in your sweet spot, you hit more professional home runs. This is usually where purpose, passion and profits meet.

> *The more you focus your time, attention and resources in your sweet spot - whether it's seeing a certain kind of patient or performing a certain medical procedure - the greater satisfaction you will experience.*

Think of how a magnifying glass focuses the sun's rays to a single point. You can carve your initials into wood with that focused ray. In a similar way, when you focus your efforts in your sweet spot, you harness the power to carve out your reputation and truly thrive.

How Does Focus Support Practice Growth?

Historically, physicians grew their practices by trying to be all things to all patients.

This is like a batter swinging at all the pitches that come their way, whether or not they are in the strike zone. The best batters wait for their favorite pitches.

Some physicians fear that narrowing their clinical scope will slow referrals. While counterintuitive, experience demonstrates that focus accelerates practice growth.

Most businesses - whether restaurants or stores or hotels - do not try to be all things to all customers; they focus and do something very, very well.

Marketing expert Seth Godin says that being average is risky. He recommends becoming remarkable. In his book The Purple Cow, Godin says, "Something remarkable is something worth talking about. Worth noticing. Exceptional. New."

Vicki took her car to a new gas station to get an oil change. When she picked it up, they had vacuumed the car. *Remarkable.*

A man needed new dress pants for an event the next day. He arrived at Nordstrom 15 minutes before closing, and walked out with hemmed pants. *Remarkable.*

A mailman noticed that an elderly woman's mail was not taken in from the previous day. Worried, he called the police. They broke down the door to find her on the floor. Had the mailman not intervened, she may well have died. *Remarkable.*

How Do Physicians Become Remarkable?

Medical organizations and individual physicians have found ways - big and small - to be remarkable.

Patients at Group Health in Seattle do not leave the medical encounter with a prescription. Instead, the prescription is entered into the computer, and patients pick up their medication from the pharmacy on their way to the car. *Remarkable.*

Virginia Mason Medical Center offers a surgical warranty for hip and knee replacements. *Remarkable.*

A dentist is passionate about working with phobic patients who have not been in the chair in a decade or more. *Remarkable.*

WHAT PUTS YOU IN A CLASS OF ONE?

There is something remarkable about you and the way you deliver medical care. The chances are good that it falls right in your sweet spot.

- Do you have a unique way of treating a medical condition?
- Do you deliver an over-the-top patient experience?
- Do you offer a unique relationship?

Here are some questions to help you identify your unique offering.

Do you create extraordinary medical outcomes?

Do you enjoy treating a specific medical condition or performing a specific procedure?

The Shouldice Clinic performs one procedure: an inguinal hernia repair. They get such extraordinary results that patients fly in from around the world to get their repair there.

In his book *Better*, Dr. Atul Gwande points out that 117 centers treat cystic fibrosis. The mean lifespan of all centers is 33 years; however, a clinic in Minnesota boasts a 47-year survival rate.

Sometimes a practice focus evolves organically. When Vicki set up her general surgical practice, she performed all of the "bread and butter" cases. Very quickly her calendar was filled with women with breast concerns.

How about you? Would you be in your sweet spot if you spent most of your days replacing mitral valves, offering advice about uncommon conditions like Grover's Disease, or helping patients at the end of their lives find more joy and experience less pain?

Do You Offer an Extraordinary Experience?

Chuck Armstrong, the former President of the Seattle Mariners, coached all of his employees: "Treat every fan as if he or she is visiting Safeco Field for the first and only time."

What level of comfort, convenience and kindness do your patients enjoy as you deliver medical care?

Does your staff see your vision and work to create this experience every day for every patient?

Do you leverage technology in new and innovative ways that improves the patient experience?

Do You Offer an Extraordinary Relationship?

The doctor-patient relationship is the foundation of the health care system. Is your practice structured in a way that you can understand what your patients want, what their health beliefs are, and why they want to achieve a given medical outcome?

Vicki has asked thousands of patients, *"What do you want in a doctor?"* Here's what they say:

- "I want a doctor who cares about me as a person."
- "I want a doctor who listens."
- "I want a doctor who treats me respectfully."
- "I want a doctor who cares what I think."
- "I want a doctor with experience with patients like me."
- "I want a doctor who will tell me the truth - kindly."
- "I want a doctor who will be there for me."
- "I want a doctor who does not judge me."
- "I want a doctor who understands that I am watching my pennies."

Patients want physicians who are authentic and present. Dr. Ed Hallowell, a child psychiatrist who treats children with ADD, openly tells the story about his personal experience with ADD.

Offering an extraordinary relationship is one of the most effective ways of being in a class of your own. How do you get in the zone?

Your focus offers clarity about what you do. It helps you strategically map out the direction of your practice's growth.

Let your innate strengths, gifts and passions guide how you do it.

Have you ever been so engrossed in an activity that time stood still? Psychologist Mihály Csíkszentmihályi describes this state as achieving *flow*. You may call it being *in the zone*.

You may find yourself in the zone when you garden, take a walk on the beach or listen to a moving piece of music.

What are you doing when you're in the zone? Are you:

- Solving a problem?
- Seeing the big picture?
- Making a discovery?
- Leading?
- Engaged in a hobby like painting, running or sailing?
- Listening to music?
- Getting things organized?
- Planning an event?
- Reading an exciting novel?
- Making something beautiful?
- Gardening?
- Exercising?
- Getting through a to-do list?

HOW TO FIND YOUR STRENGTHS AND GIFTS

You have a unique set of strengths, gifts, and passions. Paradoxically, you may look right beyond them. Things may come so easily for you when you're in your sweet spot that it's easy to dismiss your gifts.

Here are some exercises to help you identify your strength and gifts:

☑ Ask friends and colleagues, "If you could only call one person for help, under what circumstances would you call me?" or, "If I were on the cover of a magazine, what would the magazine be and what would the article be about?"

_____

_____

☑ Think about times in the past when time stood still. What were you doing? What are your hobbies?

_____

_____

☑ What compliments do you get from patients and colleagues? Please use their words.

_____

_____

☑ If you had $10 million, how would you spend your days?

_____

_____

How do others see you?
(Score = Emerging **E**, Good **G**, Breakthrough **B**)

Quality	Score	Leadership Skill	Score
Trustworthiness		Service-mindedness	
Curiosity		Listening Skills	
Optimism		Resilience	
Authenticity		Insight	
Wisdom/Mastery		Judgment	
Integrity		Charisma	

WHO ARE YOUR IDEAL PATIENTS?

Let's imagine that there is a group of patients you are here on this earth to serve. You have precisely the right tools, skills and experience to help them achieve a desired transformation. You feel passionate about helping them.

Who are these ideal patients? Here are some exercises to help you identify them.

☑ Take your daily schedule. After you see each patient, put an arrow next to their name. Point the arrow in the direction your energy goes after the visit: up, down, or the same.

☑ Now take a look at all the patients who increase your energy. What do they have in common? A personality trait? A similar life stage? Their humor?

☑ Your goal is to create an imaginary ideal patient. Some people even give this person a name.

Here are some ways to characterize your ideal patients:

- Age
- Gender
- Life stage
- Health beliefs
- Commitment to health promotion

- Willingness to adopt changes

HOW TO SPEND LESS TIME *OUTSIDE* YOUR SWEET SPOT

You have the best chance of saying yes to best-fit clients if you say no to patients and activities that drain your energy.

Byrd Tracy sings, "When mama ain't happy, ain't nobody happy."

Take a look at all the patients who drain your energy. What do they have in common? A personality trait? A similar life stage?

Identify the profile of a patient who would do better in the hands of a different doctor.

Consider culling your practice of patients who drain your energy.

WHAT ARE YOUR FINANCIAL GOALS?

Worries about money lead to "distracted doctoring." Physicians worried about money do not perform as well as financially-secure physicians.

How much money do you need to bring home each month to meet your family's minimum financial requirements? Have you factored in retirement planning, the emergency fund and your kids' educational needs?

What is your ideal revenue goal you're shooting for? Please note: you do not need to double your work to double your income. The fees from the first few patients you see each month pay your overhead; once that is met, you take home more revenue.

Clarity about your financial goals will help you make important choices. For example, you may want to donate time at a free clinic. You can use these financial numbers to make informed choices.

HOW TO IDENTIFY YOUR MOST PROFITABLE ACTIVITIES

You do not generate the same fees for all the patients you see. Some patients and procedures are more profitable than others. The profitability of each diagnostic or procedure code might offer insights that will help you craft your ideal practice.

This is where working with an outsourced billing expert becomes particularly helpful. Ask for their help in completing this analysis. Ask them to run reports that give you the revenue generated by diagnostic or procedure codes.

You may decide to continue to perform procedures, even though they are not very profitable for you; however, as you rethink your practice, you will have data to support informed choices.

WHAT ARE YOUR PERSONAL GOALS?

Work-life balance is a delicate equilibrium for physicians. What is your idea of a balanced life?

The son of a prominent surgeon describes his anger at his father for never being there. You may find that at some points personal goals are more important than financial or professional goals.

An anesthesiologist decided to cut her hours to guide her children through their teenage years.

Another physician took a leave from his practice when his father was diagnosed with a terminal illness.

Here are some questions for your consideration:

- How many times a week would you like to have family meals?
- How many of your kids' events would you like to attend?
- How much time do you devote to exercise?
- How prepared are you for life's emergencies?
- How much vacation time do you want each year?
- How many hours do you want to work each week?
- How involved are you in your community?
- How do you want to be remembered by your family, friends and patients?

HOW INSIGHTS ABOUT YOUR SWEET SPOT CAN HELP YOU

Ideally you spend as much time as possible in your sweet spot. This is when you're in the zone; this is where you find the joy.

When you're spending most of your time in your sweet spot, your work fuels you; when you spend too little time in your sweet spot, you run the risk of burning out.

Insights about how you're uniquely wired will help you design a practice that works for you.

HOW DO YOU BUILD A SUCCESSFUL PRACTICE THAT WORKS FOR YOU?

Ideally your calendar reflects your values and priorities. Is that true for you?

On a scale of 1 (low) to 5 (high), what is your satisfaction with your current level of:

- Income   ① ② ③ ④ ⑤

- Professional rewards   ① ② ③ ④ ⑤

- Work/life balance   ① ② ③ ④ ⑤

☑ Design an ideal week. How many patients would you see, and what problems would you solve?

☑ How many hours do you spend at the office, and how many at home?

☑ How are you interacting with your family? What are you doing to nourish yourself?

SUMMARY

- Don't try to be all things to all patients. Focus.
- For better practice results, spend more time in your sweet spot.
- Identify your ideal patients, your financial goals and your personal goals.

ACTION STEPS:

✓ Describe your ideal patient.

✓ Discern your financial goals.

✓ Describe your ideal week.

✓ Consider what puts you in a class of one.

2

GATHER INTELLIGENCE

Now you have a better sense of what your days would look like if you spent more time in your sweet spot.

How do you create more of those days?

Simple. You attract more of your best-fit patients and fill your calendar with sweet-spot activities.

While this is a simple plan, it can be far from easy to execute.

The key to success is understanding what your best-fit patients *really* want.

UNDERSTAND WHAT PATIENTS *REALLY* WANT

Today patients directly or indirectly drive about 80% of referrals. They decide when, where and from whom they seek health care services.

Think about the last time you flew to a medical meeting or vacation destination. You may have booked your flight on the basis of:

- Cost

- Convenience
- The overall experience
- A rewards program

Patients make choices about health care in much the same way you make choices about air travel.

You as the physician are like the pilot, navigating the route to a desired health destination. Most patients assume they will get a good medical outcome no matter where they go, just as you assume any pilot will get you to your destination safely.

You have the greatest chance of attracting your best-fit patient if you understand what patients want, when they want it and why they want it.

Here's what's most important for you to remember: patients may want very different things than you would want if you were the patient, or what you think they should want. The only way you will find out is to ask.

How did Vicki learn the hard way about wants vs needs?

Vicki made a painful $40K mistake.

One day Vicki was flying home from delivering a talk, and a passenger coded at 50,000 feet. He was traveling alone, and had absolutely no medical information on his person. Vicki and the flight attendants were able to revive him.

This episode inspired Vicki to take action and create a product she had been contemplating for many years. The Personal Health Journal is a tool that allows patients to keep track of their own version of their health stories. She invested significant resources into writing, editing and printing this product.

She was interviewed on many radio shows, offering tips to help patients collaborate more effectively with their doctors. Virtually every radio host said they loved the Personal Heath Journal, and recommended that the listeners buy the book for themselves and as a holiday gift.

Guess how many Personal Health Journals Vicki sold after appearances on 30 radio shows?

Zero.

Here's the problem. She created a product she knew patients needed; however, patients didn't want it. Patients believe that maintaining the medical record is a physician's job.

Your patients need the medical care you deliver; however, they will seek it from the physician who understands what they want, and offer it to them.

Patient-centricity - the ability to see the world through the eyes of the patient - will be key to success as we move forward.

How are you and your patients different?

It's human nature to assume that others see the world as we do, and want the same things that we want.

Physicians and patients often enter the exam room with unrecognized differences in health beliefs, perceptions and agendas. Your ability to understand what patients really want will help you:

- Attract your best-fit patients,
- Improve compliance, and
- Achieve better medical outcomes.

DIFFERENCES BETWEEN YOU AND YOUR PATIENTS

You are the medical expert; patients are medical novices. You are a native in the world of medicine, and understand the language and customs; patients are visitors.

You focus on achieving medical goals; patients' health-related behaviors are driven by their personal goals.

You manage complex medical issues on a day-to-day basis; patients face major medical issues only a handful of times in their lives.

You manage symptoms; patients live with symptoms.

You have a clear mind; patients may be frightened, in pain or medicated.

You process information in your cerebral cortex; patients process information in their limbic system.

You make medical recommendations based on clinical data; patients choose on the basis of what's most important to them. They may not take a medication because they are unwilling to live with a side effect you consider "trivial" like weight gain or nausea.

You offer patients medical leadership; patients look to you for guidance.

You measure quality of care with outcomes data; patients measure quality of care with different metrics related to their experience.

WHAT DOES "PATIENT-CENTEREDNESS" MEAN?

Physicians who run a patient-centered practice understand what it's like to walk in a patient's shoes.

Every element of their practices reflect a deep understanding of:

- **Why and when patients seek medical care**. They think creatively about how to attract patients to their practices.

- **What's important to patients.** They welcome patients, understand what frightens them and recognize the financial realities of medical care.

- **How to inspire patients to take action.** Patient-centeredness does not mean becoming a "medical short-order cook." You need not prescribe antibiotics for a kid's ear infection because the mom thinks it's a good idea. You are still there to offer medical leadership. After all, patients seek your care because of your experience, judgment and skills.

HOW TO FIND OUT WHAT YOUR PATIENTS *REALLY* WANT

There's a sure-fire way to find out. Ask them!

Howard Putnam, the CEO of Southwest Airlines, says the airline's success is based in the company's ability to see the world through the customer's eyes. He says, "We constantly surveyed our customers. After all, they were on a plane; they were a captive audience." Southwest makes choices driven by data.

How about you? Can you see the value in surveying your patients either formally or informally?

What do most patients - and referring physicians - really want?

Your patients want to be treated by physicians they trust to be the expert. How do patients know that you are an expert?

Patients are favorably impressed by:

- Seeing positive reviews of you by other patients
- Viewing patient testimonials
- Reading your blog posts
- Watching your patient educational videos
- Reading your book
- Seeing you quoted in magazines and on the news
- Following your Twitter feeds or Facebook updates
- Hearing you deliver live talks

Creating videos can be a fun and rewarding activity. Make a list of the top questions patients ask you, and record your answers. Here are some topics:

- What is cancer?
- What causes gallstones?
- How do I get my husband to take his medication as prescribed? Other video ideas:
- Demystify a medical condition.
- Summarize cutting-edge research.
- Describe a trend and predict the future.

Go to forums that attract patients like yours and see what kinds of questions they ask, then proactively offer answers. Imagine how many of your patients want to ask about sexual activity after a surgical procedure but are too embarrassed to do so.

Getting quoted in publications or interviewed on radio shows is very easy. Journalists and show producers are always looking for interesting stories. If you enjoy being a public educator, look into this. It supports expert positioning.

Demonstrate your expertise to referring physicians. Referring physicians want to send their patients to the experts, too; however, they measure expertise with different metrics than patients.

Physicians are favorably impressed when they:

- See and hear you present case series at medical meetings.

- Read your publications in peer-reviewed journals.

- Review your published outcomes data.

- Listen to webinars, podcasts or videos you create for physicians.

WHAT DO PATIENTS WANT IN ANY GIVEN ENCOUNTER?

When you enter an exam room, you are purpose-driven. Your patients may or may not share your mission. Learn more about your patients' agenda.

Ask patients, "What would you like to accomplish in our time together today?"

In general, patients want to accomplish one of four things:

- Get a diagnosis that explains their symptoms

- Get answers to their questions

- Make a plan

- Know that they are not alone, even when a cure is not possible

Ask patients, "As you consider your medical options, what's most important for you?" Some patients, for example, will do everything they can to avoid nausea. Others want to avoid taking medication.

Ask, "How has the illness impacted your life?" Or, "How will your life be better once we improve your health?" A patient with an arthritic hip may want more than pain relief; he may want to get back to the garden.

Ask, "How can we optimize the quality of each of your days?" Find out what's really important to them and then think creatively about how you can help them accomplish it. A patient may be disappointed when an acute illness keeps them from being at a family event. Maybe you can help them be there through FaceTime or Skype.

Ask, "If you were going to explain this illness or the options to your friends, what would you say?" This offers insight into their health beliefs.

Be respectful about differences in health beliefs. If your patient thinks that the rainy weather causes a flair in his bum knee, it's true for him, regardless of what the randomized prospective studies say.

You delight patients by transferring your knowledge to them in the right way, at the right time and in the right dose. The goal is not to groom a medical student. You want to help them make sense of their bodies and make good choices. Help them understand why compliance is a good choice.

Ask, "What frightens you the most about this diagnosis?" Understand patients' fears. In many cases you can offer reassurance. Gather insight into factors that could support or retard the medical plan.

The word "doctor" comes from the Latin verb *docēre*--to teach. You are a teacher. Teach in a way that allows patients to learn. Create physical models that patients can see and touch. If you have a patient with asthma, reach for a model of the lungs. Connect a straw to a balloon and ask the patient to blow it up. Then kink the straw as a metaphor for an asthma attack. Invite them to show their family at home.

Ask your patients how you're doing. Say, "On a scale of 1 to 10, how would you rate your medical care? What could we do to win a 10?"

SUMMARY

- You see the world differently than your patients do.
- Patient-centeredness is the key to practice growth.
- To grow your practice, find out what your patients really want by asking them.

ACTION STEPS:

- ✓ Survey your patients regularly.
- ✓ Gain insights into what inspires patients to take action.
- ✓ See the world through your patients' eyes.

3

YOUR MEDICAL MAKEOVER

"You only get one chance to make a first impression."

—Wisdom of the Ages

N ow you have greater clarity about who your best-fit patients are and what they want, what can you do to optimize your chances of attracting those patients and filling your days with sweet-spot activities?

WHAT IS YOUR BRAND?

When you dine at a restaurant or shop at a store or stay at a hotel, you know what kind of experience to expect. A trip to Target is different than a trip to Lord and Taylor.

Your patients, their family members and referring physicians have an impression of you and the services you offer. Let's call this impression your brand.

Is your current brand helping you - or holding your back? Is your brand consistent with every encounter?

Sometimes a mild adjustment in the way you position yourself can translate to better outcomes. For example, the California prune growers were concerned about slumping sales. They repositioned their fruit as a "dried plum" in order to distance it from images of the elderly, laxatives, and nursing homes. Sales soared.

How You Can Perform A Practice Makeover

Let's take a look at your practice through a fresh set of eyes and make sure you are putting your best foot forward.

What can your patients, referring physicians and staff expect as they work with you?

Consider what makes you different than other physicians in your medical specialty. Why would a patient choose to work with you rather than the physician down the street?

In his book *The Power of Why*, marketing guru Richard Weylman introduces the idea of a "unique value promise." Businesses distinguish themselves and grow by consistently delivering on their promises.

Here are a few examples:

- **Disneyland**: The happiest place on earth.
- **Costco**: To continually provide our members with quality goods and services at the lowest possible prices.
- **Amazon**: To build a place where people can come to find and discover anything they might want to buy online.
- **Starbucks**: To inspire and nurture the human spirit - one person, one cup and one neighborhood at a time.
- **The Ritz-Carlton Hotel**: A place where the genuine care and comfort of our guests is our highest mission.

What promise do you make to your patients, to your staff and to your referring physicians? Are you like a medical Ritz Carlton? Would you like to be the happiest medical office in your state? The absolute low-cost option?

Once you have clarity about your unique value promise, practice-building decisions follow naturally.

- If you promise compassionate care with a human touch, you know that you need to ensure that all patient encounters reflect your compassion.

- If you promise the most innovative, cutting-edge treatment, you might blog about new products and services and medical breakthroughs.

- If you build your reputation around "telling it straight," your website and all communications from your office need to be to-the-point.

Make sure that your promise is something that patients want. You could say, "We practice evidence-based medicine." Patients have no idea what that means! On the other hand, patients can and do relate to promises like "we help you get back to the activities you love."

Test your value promise with your patients.

What do you say when people ask, "What do you do?"

You can describe yourself in one of three ways:

1. **You can position yourself by your medical specialty.** The problem with this positioning is that you do not know what other people think you do. When Vicki told a child she was a general surgeon, the child replied, "So you're the person who puts warning labels on the cigarette packs!"

2. **You could offer a description of the medical conditions you treat, or your diagnostic/therapeutic tools.** The problem with this approach is that it does not separate you from the practitioners in town who do the exact same thing.

3. **You can describe yourselves in terms of the results you help patients get.** Patients come to you for a reason. They want to get from point A to point B. This is the most powerful positioning statement. Remember, behind every medical goal is a personal goal.

Here are a few examples:

- We help women optimize their heart health.

- We help weekend warriors heal their shoulder injuries and get back to the sports they love.

- We help executives perform more effectively by getting a good night's sleep.

The most magnetic positioning statement answers these three questions:

- Whom do you serve?
- What results do you help people get?
- Why is this result important?

Great positioning statements are deceptively simple. They pique the curiosity of your listener.

You know you have it when a patient calls your office and says it word for word. Once you have it, make sure that all staff members know and repeat it. Include it on your website, your email signature file and social media profiles.

Think of yourself as a change agent. You facilitate a medical transformation. Ask patients to paint before and after pictures with words. What undesired state are they trying to avoid? Ask, "What's it like living with this medical condition?" Listen for the emotion words.

Then ask, "If I had a magic wand and could instantly transform you, what would that picture look like?"

Or ask, "How do we know that treatment is successful?"

This is the before and after picture.

Your value is measured by your ability to make this transformation.

What is your physical look? Businesses make significant investments to create a visual representation of their services. They hire professionals to design logos, choose company colors and design websites, social media headers, letterhead, business cards and newsletter templates.

Many organizations have uniforms.

What about you? Here are some questions for your consideration:

What are your colors? Colors elicit an emotional response. While you can certainly choose the colors yourself, a professional can help you create the experience you want.

Do you have a logo? Have you tested it with your patients? A representation of the body part you treat could turn patients off.

Do you have a uniform, dress code or guideline about personal appearance? In general patients prefer physicians who wear white lab coats.

Do you carry your look through your letterhead, business cards, website and social media presence?

Here are some other things you need to consider when building your brand:

What do patients hear, see and smell as they walk through your front door?

- How do you welcome your patients?
- Do the front office staff greet them with a smile?
- If appropriate, do you offer them something to drink?
- Do you have uplifting reading material in your waiting room?
- Do you offer Internet access?
- Are your walls freshly painted? Is your waiting room furniture in good shape?
- Are there "medical odors" you can eliminate or mask?
- Can you add a fountain or fish tank or music that will calm patients in your waiting room?
- Do you hide frightening or intimidating pieces of equipment?

Are you engaged in social media conversations?

Are you interpreting breaking news like the change in recommendations about breast cancer screening?

Are you offering information about products and services that enhance the quality of life of patients living with a medical condition?

Are you letting people who follow you know when you have been quoted in a publication or when you spoke?

THERE IS A REASON YOU DO WHAT YOU DO

Vicki decided to become a physician when she woke from her life-saving operation. Her mission was to deliver the kind of care she wanted when she was a patient.

What is your story? Did you know you were destined to be a doctor since Kindergarten? Have you or someone you loved faced a medical crisis? What did that teach you?

As you meet with patients, share your story. Consider recording a video in which you look at the camera and tell your story to the listener.

HOW CAN SOCIAL MEDIA CONVERSATIONS HELP YOU?

However, it exposes you to potential liability. Does your medical malpractice carrier cover your social media activity? If not, look into purchasing an errors and omissions insurance policy. Create an internal policy about who will post, and what kind of content will be posted.

Treat social media like a big cocktail party. Just as you would not offer medical advice to a stranger, so too should you avoid offering diagnostic or therapeutic recommendations online.

Did a celebrity announce that they have an illness that you treat? Write about that illness in a blog post!

Do you proactively manage your online reviews? Do you follow up with patients after appointments? Do you encourage them to offer positive feedback on websites so other patients know what their experiences with you were like?

Patients are going online to evaluate your services. Set yourself up to get favorable reviews. At the end of an encounter, say, "Other patients will be interested in the kind of service we offer. What was your experience today?"

Every piece of feedback helps. If the patient offers favorable comments, say, "Would you be willing to post a comment on our Facebook page?" If they are critical, your willingness to listen may avoid an online rant.

OPTIMIZE YOUR MAGNETISM

Magnets have an interesting property; they can either attract or repel another magnet, depending on the orientation. The strength of the magnetic force is called the magnetism.

Your professional presence acts like a magnet: it can either attract the people you want to meet - or repel them.

Your goal is to optimize your magnetism so you will attract the attention of people you want to engage.

HOW TO ENHANCE YOUR MAGNETISM

Here are some tips to optimize your medical magnetism in a way that supports practice growth.

1. **Put the patient in the spotlight.** Imagine each patient encounter as a scene in a play. There's a stage with a single chair in the limelight, and more seats in the audience.

   You have two choices: you can sit on center stage and shine the limelight on yourself, or you can sit in the audience and shine the limelight on the person you serve.

   You increase your magnetism when you put the person you serve in the spotlight.

   For example, on your website you can talk about your credentials and experience. A more magnetic website talks about how you help your patients and improve their condition.

   A good way to measure this dimension of your medical magnetism is to count the number of times you say "you" and the number of times you say "I".

   You increase your magnetism by piling on the "you's."

   Begin the appointment by asking patients, "What would you like to accomplish in today's appointment?" At the end of the appointment, revisit the patient's agenda.

2. **Talk about personal outcomes rather than medical outcomes.** You have extensive experience in helping patients achieve medical goals. Find out why this medical goal is important to an individual patient. Say, "How would your life be different if

you did not have this pain?" Or, "How has this illness impacted your life?"

3. **Listen more.** Most physicians let patients speak for a short while before they direct the conversation. Invest a few more minutes into seeing the world through your patients' eyes.

4. **Tell more stories.** Numbers are the language of the thinking brain; stories are the language of the feeling brain. Emotion drives motion. Tell more stories, and quote less numbers.

5. **Say, "I care" with words and actions.** In his now famous final lecture entitled, "The Care of the Patient", Dr. Peabody spoke these moving words: "The secret of care of the patient is in caring for the patient." A profound sound bite indeed.

How do your patients know you care about them?

Let the *Five Love Languages* developed by Dr. Gary Chapman guide the way. Dr. Chapman, a minister and marriage counselor, says that we each have a native love language. Say that you care in your patient's native love language.

Words. Say to patients, "Every time I see your name on my schedule I smile; it's always a pleasure to see you."

Recognize and welcome the family caregivers who play a critical role in your patient's care.

Gifts. Gifts are a physical reminder that the recipient is important to you. They don't have to be expensive or elaborate. The best gifts are items the recipient values.

Vicki used to keep notepads in the consultation room. She would draw pictures of the gallbladder, or list three ways to sleep better. When she handed them to her patients, she was surprised to see how much they liked them! She started making a habit of giving something she wrote by hand to each of her patients.

Sometimes she would write silly prescriptions. If she knew a patient loved chocolate, she would take out her prescription pad and write "1 dark chocolate truffle PO QD. Repeat prn. Warning: this can be habit forming." Or she would tell her breast cancer patients' husbands that she had prescribed retail therapy and instruct them to take their wives to the Nordstrom's down the block.

Be contrarian and creative with your gifts. Everyone is converting to electronic medical records; give your patients a physical Personal Health Journal to store notes and records. Purchase branded items like notepads with your contact information or a fridge magnet with some health promotion tips.

Quality time. You may know someone who just wants to spend time with you. It does not matter what you're doing; the point is to do it together.

If you have a patient like this, it's time to get creative. Maybe you have a nurse or a PA enter the exam room after you're finished to address possible questions. Maybe you host a support group. Maybe you create educational videos so patients can spend time with your message.

Acts of service. Always look for ways to be helpful. If you see a patient struggling with a coat, give them a hand. Offer to make a call to a referring physician and move up their appointment. Call patients the day after a procedure and find out how they're doing. Make an audio recording of the consultation and give them a copy. (Be sure to check with your medical malpractice carrier first!)

Touch. Remember that many of your patients are touch deprived. If this is their love language, they are love deprived too. Your gentle and thorough physical exam is a way of saying "I care." Know your boundaries and potential liability when it comes to touch. Consider having a nurse in the room during an exam.

Make eye contact. Is your relationship with your computer getting in the way of your relationship with your patient? Increasingly, doctors, nurses and staff listen to patients with their ears while they look at the computer. Eye contact builds human connection.

Consider how you really want to get information in the computer. Here are a few options.

Hire a scribe - maybe a premed student - to make computer entries as you talk with patients.

Dictate as you have in the past and hire someone to do transcription.

Improve your keyboarding skills so you can keep your eyes on the patient.

Set up the office so that you can maintain eye contact as you use the keyboard.

Use an iPad or tablet. Many of the latest EHR systems are designed for the iPad, allowing you to hold it as you would a clipboard and make entries as you face the patient and look them in the eye.

Regularly elicit feedback. Say, "On a scale of one to 10, how would you rate your experience at the clinic? What can we do to earn a 10?"

Offer hope. This may be your most powerful therapeutic tool.

YOUR MAGNETIC WEBSITE

Think of your website as your professional greeter who rarely gets sick. This may be the first contact patients and information-seekers have with you.

To increase your website's magnetism, incorporate the ideas you just learned. Put the focus on how you help your clients achieve their desired outcome.

Here are some specific ways you can increase the magnetism on your website:

1. Write as if you are speaking to one person - the website visitor.
2. Create magnetic biographies that tell stories. Include photos of all of your staff members, and describe how they help patients. Consider taping a welcome video.
3. Include a call to action. Tell visitors exactly what you would like them to do next. Sign up for your newsletter? Call for an appointment?

4. Capture email addresses. Ask patients to exchange their email for an offer that has high perceived value. Get patients' permission to stay in touch.

5. Honor different learning styles by including video, audio and special reports.

6. Make information relevant and practical.

7. Make it simple.

8. Make it visual.

9. Show personality.

10. Consider having a separate part of your website for referring physicians.

11. Include patient stories.

Ask Patients for Testimonials. I know how hard it is. You think you're asking them to do you a favor, and you hate to impose, right? Here's something you may not have considered: patients are grateful for what you do for them, and they appreciate the chance to give back to you. You are actually serving them.

YOUR MAGNETIC ONLINE REPUTATION

People are going to talk about you online. You can proactively manage your online reputation.

Here are some simple steps to make your online reputation work for you:

1. Claim your free online listings. At the minimum set up free profiles on Google, Yelp and Bing Places and Yellow Pages.

2. Google yourself. See what your patients and referring physicians see when they look you up.

3. Proactively manage your online reviews. Patients are going online to evaluate your services. Set yourself up to get favorable reviews. At the end of an encounter, say, "Most patients want to know what kind of experience they can expect at our office. Would you

be willing to help them by completing an online evaluation or taping a video describing your experience?"

4. Regularly follow up with patients so their feedback comes to you - and is not vented in an online rant.

5. Set up Google alerts for medical conditions, procedures you perform and the problems for which you offer solutions.

All Patient Feedback is Helpful. Every piece of patient feedback helps. If the patient offers favorable comments say, "Would you be willing to put that on an online evaluation?" If they are critical, your willingness to listen may avoid an online rant.

A WEEK OF HEALTHY HABITS

Try doing this for 4 weeks - 28 days.

Measuring Monday. Look at your schedule for the upcoming week and notice which activities get you excited and which make you feel drained.

Talking Tuesday. Begin each conversation with something positive. Instead of beginning a patient encounter by asking what the problem is, ask, "What's the best thing that happened this week?"

Wakeup Wednesday. Pay attention to the things that are going right.

Thank-you Thursday. Find at least one person to thank. It's especially fun if this person is normally unseen and unappreciated - the person who cleans your office, or who takes your money at the hospital cafeteria. Tell them specifically how they make your life better. Consider writing a thank-you note to someone who referred a patient or served as a mentor or a source of inspiration.

Feedback Friday. Ask one person, "How am I doing as your doctor/employer/partner/parent/child?" Then ask, "How could I do better?"

Saturday Relief. Consider taking a break from the to-do list. Turn off your computer and park your cell phone in a drawer. Be present with your family. Read a book. Do something that recharges you.

Dreaming Sunday. Spend 10 minutes thinking about the things you would love to do and have always wanted to do.

SUMMARY

- You only have one chance to make a first impression; make the most of your opportunities!
- You can enhance your medical magnetism and improve your ability to engage patients and referring physicians.
- Your positioning statement, website, marketing materials and online presence have magnetic qualities.

ACTION STEPS:

- ✓ Craft a memorable, repeatable positioning statement.
- ✓ Measure and improve the magnetism of your verbal, written and online messages.
- ✓ Start posting patient testimonial videos.

4

PAVE PATHS TO YOUR DOOR

"Satisfied patients stay; delighted patients deliver referrals."

-Vicki Rackner

You need a steady stream of new patients to run a thriving medical practice.

Even the most successful businesses like Apple invest to attract new customers.

HOW TO BUILD NETWORKS OF REFERRALS

Developing and maintaining a steady stream of new patients is particularly important if you are:

- Beginning a practice
- Developing a focus in your current practice
- Seeing shifting referral patterns as your current sources of referrals retire or sell their practices

Here are four steps to help you accelerate your practice growth by generating more patient referrals. This means grooming more SENDERS - people who send patients your way.

STEP #1: DELIGHT YOUR PATIENTS

When it comes to practice-building, satisfied patients stay; delighted patients deliver referrals.

Furthermore, delighted patients get back to the SENDER and say good things about you; this supports further referrals.

Here are some ideas that will help you create an extraordinary experience that delights your patients.

Treat your patients as the distinguished guests of honor they are. And do it in a way that works for your practice. You want office efficiency, but not at the expense of practice growth.

Some ideas that delight your patients may inconvenience your staff or cost a few dollars. It's more efficient, for example, to let your calls go to voicemail. However, voice mail cannot send you referrals; delighted patients can. You are making an investment to acquire a new patient that has life-long value for your practice.

Create a sense of welcome. Think back to a time when you went someplace new and a stranger helped you feel right at home.

Vicki walked into the radio studio to tape a public service announcement and saw a note behind the receptionist. "Warm 106.9 welcomes Dr. Rackner." That simple gesture set the tone for the entire experience.

The way you welcome patients to your practice - whether it's when they call or walk through the front door - can build a bridge to delighted patients or build walls.

Vicki referred a patient to an excellent neurologist. Her patient liked the physician but refused to go back because the front office staff were so rude to her.

Hire the right staff. Think of your front office staff as "Ambassadors of Welcome." Hire people who have a warm smile and a pleasing voice. Value them and respect them. Ask them for their ideas about how to improve the patient experience.

One HR executive said, "I can teach most people almost any technical task; what I cannot teach is how to be friendly."

Encourage staff to place a small mirror next to the phone; the smiles on their faces comes through in their voice. Coach staff to use the caller's name. Stagger lunches so that you have a live person answering the phone during busy call times.

> "Never go to a doctor whose office plants have died."
>
> *Erma Bombeck*

Fill the waiting room with uplifting reading material. Your patients have plenty of access to newspapers and fear-based magazines. Let your office be an oasis of hope and optimism.

If you create educational videos, offer a place to view them.

Say hello with a name and a smile. Coach your staff to make eye contact and offer a smile as they welcome patients.

Have a name conversation. At the first visit coach your staff to clarify name preferences. Say, "Names are important to us, and we want to get it right. Feel free to call me Sally. A few people call the doctor Dr. Rackner, but most call her Dr. Vicki. What name do you prefer? Mr. Evans? Paul?" Record this critical piece of information in the patient record. Include phonetics (MEIR; pronounce like "mayor").

> "Remember that a person's name is to that person the sweetest and most important sound in any language."
>
> *Dale Carnegie*

Consider including a photo in the medical record. It circumvents the confusion when two patients have the same name and prevents medical mishaps. Say, "We always want to make sure we're talking to the right person, so we have pictures on file."

Begin and end the physician encounter with a handshake. It builds trust at the beginning of the encounter and seals an agreement about next steps at the end.

Get groomed. Patients want medical staff to dress formally. According to a poll with the AMA, 65% preferred their doctors in white coats. Over half preferred that their doctors didn't wear blue jeans.

Consider some basic uniform for the staff. Maybe it's a shirt or jacket with your logo on.

Run on time. Here are three good reasons:

- First, it shows your patients that you value your time
- Second, it builds trust
- Third, it promotes referrals

If you're running late, or patients are put on hold as a matter of routine, the perception is that you are already too busy.

STEP #2: CREATE YOUR REFERRAL MAP

How do patients find their way to you?

If you're like most practices, about 80% of your referrals come from 20% of the SENDERS.

Here are some common SENDERS:

- Patients
- Physicians
- Your employees and volunteers
- Family members of your patients
- Nurses
- Internet searches
- Clergy
- Audience members of your speaking engagements
- Viewers of media appearances

Understand who your SENDERS are.

THREE SOURCES OF UNLIMITED REFERRALS

Medical professionals, whether referring physicians, through the ER or via other health care providers.

Family, friends and fans who know you, like you and trust you.

- Your delighted patients and their family members
- Members of your community
- People in your social circles, like the parents of your kids' soccer team members
- People you hire, like your hairdresser
- Alumni

Information-seekers who go online, read publications or attend courses to find solutions to pressing medical problems.

Each physician has a unique mix of referral sources based on their practice setting, medical specialty and temperament.

Here's what Vicki learned when she informally surveyed physicians at a surgical meeting:

Academic physicians tend to get most of their new patients from referring physicians. They rely heavily on their institution's brand strength to generate referrals.

Community physicians performing bread-and-butter cases leverage their personal and professional relationships.

Physicians with focused practices (breast surgery, bariatric procedures and plastic surgeons) generate almost 100% of their patient referrals by connecting directly with them. The pharmaceutical industry calls it direct-to-consumer marketing.

Campaigns to generate referrals from the three sources will be different.

Understand patients' triggers for action. Gain insight into what propels patients to pick up the phone and call your office. Then, think creatively about how you can put yourself in front of these patients.

If you are trying to grow a breast imaging center, for example, you know that often the diagnosis of breast cancer in a friend, or the illness of a family member inspires patients to schedule the overdue mammogram.

A breast center could launch a campaign to encourage their patients to spread the word about the importance of screening mammograms. Maybe you distribute buttons that say, "Friends don't let friends skip mammograms." Maybe you print up postcards your patients can give to their friends inviting their friends to get mammograms. Maybe you offer a 5% discount for friends of your patients.

Understand where patients go for help before they call you. Do they consult with Dr. Google? If so, what words did they put into the search field?

Do they call other professionals or buy certain products? When you know the answers to these questions, think creatively about how you can put yourself in front of these patients.

STEP #3: ADOPT THE REFERRAL MINDSET

When Vicki speaks, she often asks audience members, "Do you think that asking for referrals is an effective way to get more patients?" Almost 100% say, "Yes."

Then she asks the second question. "How often do you ask for referrals?" The most common answer is "Never." When she was running her own surgical practice, she fell into this group.

When Vicki asks physicians why they do not ask for referrals; here's what they say:

- "I shouldn't have to ask for referrals; if I do a good job, my patients will automatically tell their friends."
- "It's unprofessional to ask for referrals. I'll look like a used car salesman."
- "I don't want to impose on my patients."
- "I get so busy I forget to ask."
- "Asking for referrals makes my patients uncomfortable."

- "Asking for referrals makes me uncomfortable."
- "Nobody at the office likes doing it."

If you think that you're imposing, asking for a favor or otherwise alienating people, you avoid the behavior!

There's another way of thinking about referrals that leads to much better results.

EMBRACE THE SPIRIT OF SERVICE

You chose a career in medicine to serve others. And while there are other doctors in your community who have your training, you provide your patients with a unique experience. There's a group of patients out there who are best served when they find their way to you. If you are dedicated to serving those patients, you must give them the opportunity to find you.

You are not asking your patients for favors; you're asking for the opportunity to make an impact in a bigger way.

Referrals are not about you or about the person you ask for the introduction; they're about the people you can serve.

Challenge your assumptions about your patients' mindset.

Many fear that the request for introductions places a burden on patients.

Consider this. Your patients are grateful for your care. They want to give back. When you ask for introductions, you're telling them exactly what you would most appreciate: the chance to help others. This is like telling a friend what you would like to do on your birthday.

Moreover, we as a species are wired to share resources. Sharing what you know is a form of social currency.

Challenge your assumptions about asking for help.

Many medical professionals resist asking others for help; they fear it's a demonstration of weakness that will compromise their stature.

Your SENDERS will appreciate the chance to help!

A Personal Story

When Vicki began her speaking career, she was very nervous before she went onstage. What if she lost her train of thought? What if she couldn't answer audience members' questions?

When she thought about her performance, her anxiety shot up.

Then a mentor suggested she take the focus off of herself and put it where it should be - on the audience members. What were their needs?

When she thought about how she could serve the audience, she calmed down and gave her best.

Referrals are not about you; they're about your best-fit patients who need you.

Step #4: Create A Culture of Referrals

You can plant the seeds of referrals at many points in the relationship with your SENDERS - the people who send you patients.

Create scripts that all your staff members can practice and say by rote. Let's say a patient offers a compliment. Say, "Thank you. That is so kind. Our intention is to provide such extraordinary service that you tell all your family and friends about us."

Consider launching a bold mission, and invite others to join you. "We're on a mission to ensure that kids learn how amazing their bodies are! Will you help us by letting kids and parents know we have educational videos on our website?"

Offer clues about when to make referrals. Share these clues with your patients so they know the trigger for an appropriate referral.

If you're an orthopedic surgeon, say, "If you see someone rubbing their knee when they play golf - or give up the game all together - have them give us a call. We're here to help people enjoy the sports they love."

If you're a sleep doctor, say, "If you see someone yawning at lunch or nodding off at a meeting, invite them to get our special free report about sleep."

Keep meticulous records of referrals. You want to know EXACLY how patients found their way to your door. Look for patterns.

Thank SENDERS. Send a handwritten thank-you note. Of course, HIPAA regulations mandate that you must not share the patient's name. You can say, "We saw a new patient in our office today who came here at your recommendation. We just want to let you know how grateful we are to have your trust."

Ask referred patients to thank the SENDER. Say, "Because of HIPAA regulations, I cannot tell the person who made the referral that you were here today; however, please get back to them and let them know what your experience with our office was like."

Before and after pictures. If you've ever watched a makeover program, you know the power of before and after pictures. Think about how you can harness this power in your own practice.

Some medical specialties like cosmetic surgery and orthodontic care lend themselves to physical pictures. Give patients copies of their before and after pictures. Some practices even make customized business cards. The front would look like your business card; the back is your patient's before and after picture. You can buy 250 cards for bargain rates.

Most medical practices will need to create verbal pictures of the transformation during medical care. "Do you remember the first time you came in? You were scared and confused. You didn't know what choices were right. Now look at you. You're smiling, spending time with your family and back at work. What a transformation!"

Create educational materials. Your patients may not know if you would be a good fit for their friends, relatives and colleagues. If you create educational videos, your patients can advise that people watch the videos, and decide for themselves if they want to become your patient.

Read dating books and visit dating sites. Let's say you decided it was time to find your soul mate. The chances are good that you would tell your friends and relatives exactly what you were looking for.

Think of each relationship you have with a patient as a medical marriage. Your search for your ideal patients can follow along the same lines. Tell patients exactly what you are looking for; that would make your patients the matchmakers.

PRACTICE-BUILDING IS RELATIONSHIP-BUILDING

Invest in relationships with the people who send you patients. Educate them. Offer them value. Make it easy for them to identify patients you treat and the circumstances that would trigger a referral.

To generate more referrals and build your practice, serve the people who send you patients.

Tell stories rather than quote facts. Let's say you want to persuade primary physician SENDERS to refer more patients to your pain clinic or hospice. You could say, "Patients under our care experience a 30% reduction in overall pain scores." Or you could tell the story of a fractured family reconciling. You have a much better chance of persuading with the story.

Listen to great storytellers. Watch TED videos at **www.TED.org**. Hear great speakers.

Tell more stories at the dinner table, with your staff and with your SENDERS.

Post a bulletin board where people can share stories.

Focus on people who "get it" vs people who don't. Some referring physicians simply cannot see the difference between treating patients themselves and referring them to you. Many frustrated staff ask, "How do we help them understand? They just don't seem to get it."

Your time is better invested in connecting with people who "get it" rather than converting people who don't.

WHAT IS THE KEY TO SUCCESS IN MEDICAL PRACTICE?

The best way to get what you want is to help others get what they want.

Your SENDERS may include referring physicians, patients, nurses or your neighbor. Each SENDER wants different things.

Your ability to see the world through your SENDERS' eyes and help them become more successful will accelerate your practice growth.

As you think of a person with whom you want to connect, consider key questions:

- What are their unmet needs?
- What keeps them up at night?
- What would you say to this person if they were a friend or relative?

Remember the main point from the psychology of persuasion: **Emotions drive motion.**

WHAT DO REFERRING PHYSICIANS WANT?

1. They want to be appreciated by their patients.

You want patients to go back to their referring physician raving about you. As you see patients and delight them, say, "Please let Dr. Jones know what you thought about the care here."

2. They want to be appreciated by you.

Launch a "growth through gratitude" campaign. Send one handwritten thank-you note a day to individuals who send you patients. You'll build your practice for the cost of a postage stamp.

You will most likely find that most of your referrals come from a small percentage of physicians. Do you send them gifts? If their love language is gift-giving, a thoughtful, personal gift is a nice touch. If you know a physician loves airplanes and you see a coffee table book, purchase it for them!

3. They want to experience mastery.

Create an e-newsletter in which you share your clinical pearls, overturn myths and educate physicians about recent developments in your specialty.

WHAT DO PATIENTS WANT?

1. Patients want to be remembered.

Send a birthday greeting. This is a very easy way to cultivate an ongoing relationship.

2. Patients want you to hold them in high regard.

Say to them, "We so appreciate patients like you. We're grateful to the people who refer people like you to our practice! Feel free to let others know about our services. We're always happy to see new patients."

3. Patients want a way to express their gratitude.

Give them the chance to give back. Ask if they'd be willing to talk to other patients. Invite them to write a testimonial or tell their story on video. You're not troubling them; you may be delighting them. Think about how good you feel when you're given the chance to give.

WHAT DO NURSES WANT?

Nurses want to feel connected.

Nurses are team players by temperament; however, visiting nurses in particular often feel alone in managing complex problems. Let them know they can count on you. Ask them what they would like to learn about and offer a CME course.

WHAT DO FAMILY CAREGIVERS WANT?

Family caregivers are your therapeutic allies to enhance medication compliance, decrease hospital readmissions and improve clinical outcomes. They also direct referrals from behind the scenes. They're talking with their friends. They're searching the Internet. They want the best care for their loved ones, but they don't want to work with strangers. Give them a chance to get to know you.

1. They want information.

Write articles or create videos that answer questions family caregivers ask.

2. They want support.

Host a caregiver support group. You can either hold it in your office or let people join by phone or Skype.

3. **They want to be included.**

Ask how they're doing when they bring their loved ones in for appointments.

WHAT DO SMALL BUSINESSES WANT?

Small businesses are the engines that drive our economy. If you can help local businesses get new customers, everyone benefits.

1. **They want more customers.**

Ask local businesses about products or services your patients would want to know about.

2. **They want to add value to their customer experience.**

They offer special or discounted services to their customers. Give businesses the chance to give your patients a discount.

SUMMARY

- You have a unique referral map.
- Satisfied patients stay; delighted patients deliver referrals.
- Adopt a referral mindset.
- The best way to get what you want is to give others what they want.

ACTION STEPS:

✓ For the next 30 days, ask each patient how and why they found their way to you. Get as specific as possible.

✓ Ask your patients, "How did you get our name?"

   If they say, "My doctor's office," ask, "Who at the office gave you my name?"

   If they say, "A friend," ask, "How did your friend know us? Did we treat them?"

If they say, "An Internet search," ask, "What words did you type in the search bar?"

For new patients, ask, "What made you call us today rather than last week or last month?"

✓ **Create a database of referral sources** so you can follow trends (case manager vs visiting nurse vs assisted living). This is extremely important, because you want to develop ongoing relationships with existing SENDERS.

✓ **Build a referral map.** Identify the paths patients take to find you. Get a piece of paper and draw a wheel with lots of spokes. Put yourself at the center; each spoke represents your relationship with a SENDER.

✓ List 5 major SENDERS

1. _____
2. _____
3. _____
4. _____
5. _____

✓ Review your website and promotional material. How often does the spotlight shine on you, and how often does it shine on the people you serve?

✓ Coach everyone in your organization so they are all skilled at communicating your value. Make sure every single person associated with your organization knows what to say when someone asks, "What do you do?" The very best approach is to engage the listener with a problem. "Have you ever known someone who lives with chronic pain, and no one seems to listen or understand? We help these people have more good days and recapture joy."

✓ Write down 3 "out-of-the-box" ideas.

1. _____
2. _____
3. _____

5

LAUNCH MARKETING CAMPAIGNS THAT WORK

How do you avoid being the best-kept secret in town?

That's where marketing comes in.

Marketing is nothing more than engaging people in conversation. To be heard above the noise, you want to deliver the right message to the right person at the right time.

You then want to persuade your conversation partner to take action.

And remember, people like to interact with people they know, like and trust.

Launching a marketing campaign is much like giving a terrific gift:

1. You identify the gift recipient.
2. You select a gift that the recipient wants. The biggest mistake is giving the gift that you want.
3. You wrap the gift.
4. You deliver the gift.

THE FOUR STEPS TO AN AWESOME MARKETING CAMPAIGN

We call these the elements of the "Golden Triangle."

1. Identify the audience of the marketing campaign. Are you reaching out to family, friends and fans? Information-seekers? Power partners? You will deliver the same message in very different ways and with different language. When you have clarity about whom you are trying to engage, you are most likely to get their attention.

2. Craft an offer. This means delivering something the recipient *really* wants. You may know what they need. However, keep in mind Vicki's $40K mistake. What do patients really want to know? What do your referring physicians really want to know? What question are information-seekers really searching for?

3. Package your intellectual property. You may decide to write an article, create educational videos or deliver a seminar. Even better, package the same intellectual property in all of the above ways!

4. Distribute your content. Now that you have packaged this content, it's time to get it out there.

You want the recipient to say, "Wow, you really 'get me!'"

Always offer a call to action. Think of marketing as the process of engaging people in conversation, and selling as the process of inspiring your conversation partner to take action. Every marketing campaign should offer both. Tell your conversation partner exactly what you want them to do.

Here are some calls to action:

1. Call your office to set up a complimentary appointment with you.
2. Get your brochure or special report.
3. Read your book.
4. Sign up to be on your mailing list.

THE THREE TARGETS OF AN EFFECTIVE MARKETING CAMPAIGN

1. **Family friends and fans.** These are people who already know, like and trust you. This is the source of "low-hanging fruit."

Reaching out to members of this group and informing them of your value proposition is the fastest, easiest and most effective way to generate more patient referrals.

2. **Information-seekers.** Patients and their loved ones actively seek information about a specific medical condition or a specific problem for which they seek a solution. If you position yourself as an expert and create intellectual property, patients can and will find you.

Here are some activities that support expert positioning:

- Blog
- Create educational videos
- Get quoted in the media
- Write a book
- Give lectures

Patients want to be assured that you can help them get their desired results.

Your colleagues, on the other hand, are much more interested in your certifications.

3. **Power Partners.** These are people who influence the choices of your best-fit patients. Your power partners may or may not be healthcare professionals. Ideally, they:

- Come into regular contact with your best-fit patients
- Have the respect of those patients
- Influence patients' choices

Invest some time here. Be creative. Ask yourself, "When a patient has the problem I solve, with whom do they interact?" Examples:

Physician/Doctor	Result	Power Partners
Sports Medicine Specialist	Optimizing athletic performance	Coaches, trainers, massage therapists

| Rheumatologist with a special interest in MS | Optimize the quality of life for patients living with MS | MS support groups Businesses that sell products to people living with MS |
| Orthodontist | Helping brides get picture-perfect smiles | Wedding planners Bridal shops |

THREE TYPES OF MARKETING CAMPAIGNS THAT WORK

Educational marketing. These are campaigns in which you engage patients and SENDERS by offering high-value educational content. You can do this through writing, speaking, video creation, podcasts or seminars. This is an excellent fit for physicians. After all, the word doctor comes from the Latin root meaning "teacher." Educational marketing supports expert positioning.

Relationship marketing. These are campaigns in which you build relationships with SENDERS. You can hire professional relationship-builders that go out on your behalf and build strategic relationships.

Community marketing. These are campaigns in which you become the architect of a community. Maybe you create a virtual community through social media. Maybe you create a community of people dedicated to bringing service dogs to hospitals. Maybe you form a group of women that knit.

There are three time scales for results.

Of course, it will take some time before you see the results of your marketing.

Short-term. You can see very rapid results when you launch campaigns to family, friends and fans.

Medium-term. Building relationships with power partners takes time. However, it's time well spent.

Long-term. Packaging your intellectual property and getting it out there can potentially get you rapid results. However, think of it as the long haul. A patient may be on your mailing list for months before they pick up the phone and call you.

EXAMPLES OF POWERFUL MARKETING CAMPAIGNS

Family - Friends - and - Fans Educational Campaign

Go to people who already know, like and trust you and say, "You may not know this about me, but I'm on a mission to decrease the suffering from lupus. If you know anyone who would like to learn more about lupus, please invite them to go to my website and sign up for my video series."

Schmoozing - in - the - Doctor's - Dining - Room Relationship Campaign

Let's say you want more referrals from the primary care physician at your institution. Eat lunch there when they do! If they talk about baseball, learn something about baseball so you can join the conversation. Remember, our brains are wired with mirror neurons. The statement "I like you" really means, "I'm like you. I see part of myself reflected in you."

Information - Seeker Seminar Campaign

Let's say you and your multi-disciplinary team wanted to treat more pancreatic cancer patients. You could launch multiple campaigns. A physician who is media trained may be interviewed on the radio or TV about what's new in the treatment of pancreatic cancer. You could promote a fundraiser in which the proceeds go to pancreatic cancer research. You could present case studies at medical meetings. You could also speak at the oncology nursing association. You could have a Facebook page.

Be quoted. Getting quoted in the press is very easy once you know the ropes. People who host social media conversations are always on the lookout for great content they can curate. Radio hosts and editors are always looking for interesting stories and interesting guests. Invest in media coaching, and learn to communicate in sound bites.

Now you have a picture of what you would like to do, the next question is how to get there.

Which marketing campaigns will work for you?

MADE-TO-ORDER MEDICAL MARKETING CAMPAIGNS

Here's an easy way to create campaigns. It works like a deli sandwich order form. Choose one item from section A (the expert content you will deliver), section B (the audience to whom you speak) and section C (content delivery vehicle) to create programs and products.

A. Content
    i. Disease management
    ii. Colleague support and education
    iii. Peer support and education
    iv. Caregiver support and education
    v. Patient support and education
    vi. Strategies/products to enhance the quality of life.

B. Audiences
    i. Primary care practitioners and specialty practitioners
    ii. Current and former patients
    iii. Family caregivers
    iv. Visiting nurses
    v. Eldercare providers
    vi. Local businesses
    vii. Professional organizations
    viii. Peers beginning their careers
    ix. Service organizations
    x. Religious groups
    xi. Journalists
    xii. Internet information seekers

C. Content delivery vehicles
    i. Written word (articles/brochures/books)
    ii. Video
    iii. Courses (live, self-study)
    iv. Support groups
    v. A live experience/event

vi. Social media outreach

vii. Media exposure

viii. Teleseminar

ix. Webinar

x.   Podcasts

Instructions: Choose one from column A, one from column B and one from column C. There are hundreds of options.

There are so many choices. Where do you begin? You have three basic strategies:

1 **Cast your net wider.** Do more of what's already working. If you get referrals from the nail salon, approach more nail salons in your area.

2 **Dig deeper.** Maybe you want to focus on a specific procedure or medical condition.

3 **Try something new.** Step out of your comfort zone. Make a radio appearance. Write a brochure. Take on a leadership position.

You do not have to do all the work yourself. You do not have to create all your own content; you can offer the content of others. There are people who can offer skills you need to take on new projects, like creating audio CDs, videos, reports, etc.

If you're drawn to an idea, there are people who can help you make it happen. Check out www.fiverr.com.

TEST AND MEASURE

Here is the biggest piece of advice for launching successful campaigns: test and measure! You invest resources into marketing campaigns. What is the return on your investment? Have metrics that you can objectively observe. The ultimate question is, "How many new patients came from that marketing campaign?

Sometimes it's hard to say. Campaigns can work synergistically. First a "patient prospect" hears you deliver a seminar. They get an e-newsletter from you once a month. Then they hear you interviewed on the radio and finally decide it's time to take action. Each piece of intellectual property that you put out there increases your chances of getting known. Regular contributions work best.

Should You Advertise?

Marketing and advertising are different. Advertising says with words and actions "Let me tell you all about me." Marketing says with words and actions, "Let's talk about you."

Many physicians advertise on radio and TV. Just today we heard a radio ad for a center that treats back pain. It said something like, "Do you have back pain? Come see us. You'll be treated with state-of-the-art care."

What if instead the physician were a guest on a radio show talking about recent developments in the treatment of back pain?

Today's information overload means people have gotten better at ignoring unwanted messages, including ads and commercials. They pay closest attention to messages about them or about something important to them. You are much more likely to influence when turning the spotlight on SENDERS and making them the focus of your conversation.

Marketing accelerates practice growth more quickly than advertising in the post-Google era. It's also more cost effective.

Advertising vs. Marketing

When you advertise, you typically offer the same message to most audiences - one size fits all.

Practice-building in the Pre-Google World	Practice-building in the Post-Google World
You advertise.	You market.
You invite primary care doctors to your open house.	You invite primary care doctors to your content-rich webinars.
You offer facts.	You tell stories.

Practice-building in the Pre-Google World	Practice-building in the Post-Google World
You run ads in the newspaper.	You're quoted in the newspaper.
You buy radio air time and run ads.	You're the guest interviewed on the radio show.
You tell others about your credentials on your website.	You offer patient testimonials on your website.

If you invest in advertising, consider social media advertising or direct mail. Then measure the ROI.

Vicki remembers starting her practice. She purchased a newspaper ad. When it didn't generate any interest, the newspaper told her that she needed to buy more ads! (She found other ways to build her practice.)

Summary

- Marketing is the act of engaging people in conversation; selling is the act of inspiring people to take action.

- Launching marketing campaigns is like giving the perfect present.

- Advertising puts you in the spotlight; marketing puts your conversation partner in the spotlight.

ACTION STEPS:

✓ Look at your best 20 patients, and identify the marketing campaign that attracted them to you.

✓ Make a list of the marketing campaigns you launched last year.

✓ Calculate the investment for each campaign, and determine the return.

6

LET'S TALK ABOUT MONEY

If you have any friends who run businesses, you know that they have a different relationship with money than you do. A recent episode of the reality TV show, *Shark Tank*, offers insights about the differences.

A doctor entrepreneur entered the Shark Tank asking for a $3 million investment to grow his medical device company. He painted the picture of an ideal investment opportunity, complete with an innovative product, a huge proven market and $10 million in sales.

As we listened, we thought, "He could get a five-Shark deal!"

However, things quickly fell apart during Q&A. Here are snippets from the exchange sparked by the Sharks' inquiries about his sales:

Doctor: "We could be making quite a bit of money if I wanted to. I'm not all that interested in the money. It's a tool I use to hire people."

Lori Greiner: "You're not interested in making money?"

Doctor: "It's not my motivation. Medical training is very important. It's a way of saving lives. "

Kevin O'Leary: "What about profits? Do you care about this?"

Doctor: "I will at some point."

By the end of the pitch, four Sharks were out. Robert Herjavec decided to invest, and the deal fell through for undisclosed reasons several days later.

Money is a tool to help you get what you want too. However, without money your hands might be tied behind your back.

If you want to serve in a big way, we must talk about money. We know, it doesn't come easy!

WHY DO PHYSICIANS AVOID CONVERSATIONS ABOUT MONEY?

Here are three reasons why most physicians shy away from conversation about money.

1. **The culture of medicine.** Just as the government calls for the separation of church and state, medical ethics calls for a separation between patient care and a patient's ability to pay. Physicians are expected to make medical choices blinded to financial concerns. As a practicing physician Vicki often thought that ordering medical services was like ordering a restaurant meal off a menu without any prices. It's no wonder health care costs spiraled out of control!

2. **Low financial literacy.** Physicians get no formal training in business or financial management in medical school or residency. Physicians are required to make ongoing investments in medical education; most have a strong preference for content that helps them improve patients' health rather than their own financial health.

3. **Awareness of their vulnerability.** In nature, an animal is either predator or prey. Physicians experience themselves as financial prey. They are the targets of frequent pitches by people who want to work with the "rich doctors." They intuitively know they do not have the financial savvy to assess the true risks and merits of

business opportunities. They fall prey to DDDs - dumb doctor deals.

THREE REASONS YOU MUST OVERCOME THE TABOO ABOUT MONEY

1. Patients want to talk about medical expenses. They have more financial skin in the game.
2. We practice medicine in an era of greater financial transparency.
3. If you are worried about meeting your expenses, you are siphoning attention away from patient care.

> *The bottom line is this: if you want to serve your patients, you must meet your financial goals.*

An entrepreneurial physician contacted Vicki to inquire about her coaching services. He had a proven system for empowering patients to resolve a complex medical issue, and wanted help launching a multi-disciplinary team that delivered innovative services.

Vicki could feel his clinical passion. Then she started asking questions about the economic viability of this venture.

He told her that he was uncertain whether the insurance company would pay for his services and that patients in his area were simple unwilling to pay cash for medical services.

He also could not pay his mortgage.

If you do not have a financially-viable practice, you have a hobby.

WHAT IS YOUR RELATIONSHIP WITH MONEY?

You have beliefs about money - how to acquire it, how to spend it, and whether you are worthy of wealth.

Very simply, you were most likely raised with a mindset of abundance or a mindset of scarcity. You will bring those beliefs into adulthood by default, and recreate their childhood financial reality.

These beliefs can be reprogrammed (see Appendix A). You can rebuild your relationship with money just like you build a relationship with a friend.

How Do You Respond to Financial Pain?

As Vicki treated patients, she noticed patterns in the way patients responded to physical pain. She identified "5 pain personalities."

People respond to physical pain in much the same way they respond to financial pain, so here they are:

The Strong Stoic. A sturdy Scandinavian patient said, "You needed to be near death's door before Mother called the doctor. Sure, money was tight. I think the real reason we didn't go to doctor was pride. Although Mother never said it, we knew that being healthy and being tough were sources of pride. Illness and pain were shameful conditions that were hidden."

Strong stoics may try to manage their own finances even when they are over their heads. If you are married to a Strong Stoic, emphasize the courage and the strength of character to seek advice and focus on the return to financial health.

The Worried Well. Think of the multi-millionaire haunted by the irrational fear of becoming homeless. Another name for this person is the "financial hypochondriac."

These are intelligent people who hear about a new financial ill on the news, and recognize that they have several of the symptoms - and maybe they have this diagnosis! They know just enough to be dangerous.

The Worried Well do best with regularly scheduled reality checks. Just as a broken watch is right twice a day, financial ills really can strike!

The Ostrich. We all need a healthy dose of denial to get on with our days. However, denial can go overboard and threaten financial health.

If you partner is an Ostrich, your most effective strategy is to understand their reality, then offer an alternative point of view. Support this with the authority of the opinion or story of a doctor colleague.

The Victim. Some people experience themselves as victims of external circumstances. Furthermore, they're powerless to change their reality. Victims often dismiss ideas that could empower them.

If you try to help a Victim, expect challenges. Their words say they want to achieve financial health, but their actions say something quite different.

The Ideal. The ideal gets engaged, makes proactive choices and has a well-calibrated intuition.

Knowing your pain personality is like knowing your tennis swing. If you observe that the swing pulls to the right, you make adjustments to get the ball where you want it to go.

Similarly, insights into your pain personality help uncover financial conflicts. Imagine a Strong Stoic married to a Worried Well.

Which of these ideas best align with your own beliefs about wealth?

"I'm entitled to wealth." You and your family made tremendous sacrifices to answer this call to medical service. A high income is part of the package.

"Look at me!" This physician wants to maintain the appearance of success.

"I'm embarrassed." Many physicians wonder why they make more money than others.

"Mother Theresa took a vow to poverty; I should, too." This physician does not feel worthy of wealth.

Treat Money with Respect

You are more likely to attract more money into your life if you treat it with respect. Put the bills in your wallet facing the same way. Keep a change jar. For a month, keep track of every penny you spend.

Talk with Patients about Finances

As you speak with patients about their medical options, ask, "How do your finances impact your medical choices?"

Talk with Your Children about Finances

Help your children develop a healthy relationship with money. Speak with them about the responsibility that accompanies wealth. Help them manage their own money.

SUMMARY

- For physicians, money is the ultimate taboo topic.
- You can no longer afford to avoid conversations about money.
- You can improve your relationship with money.

ACTION STEPS:

- ✓ Explore your relationship with money.
- ✓ Identify your pain personality.
- ✓ Initiate conversations with your patients about medical finances.

7

HOW MONEY FLOWS INTO AND OUT OF YOUR PRACTICE

Managing the financial health of your practice is much like managing the health of your patients. You watch and measure pertinent numbers.

In the ICU, you measure your patients' input and output.

In a similar way, it's important to watch the money that flows in and out of your practice. Business people call this the *cash flow*.

How do you improve cash in-flow?

1. Identify profitable activities
2. Address billing practices

IDENTIFY PROFITABLE ACTIVITIES IN YOUR PRACTICE NOW

What are the activities that go on in your office each day that you can consider profitable? (Of course we are only referring to financial profitability, not whether or not it is of value to you, such as job satisfaction or patient well-being.)

Seeing patients is obviously a profitable activity. Some patients, not all of them. As mentioned earlier, seeing the patients that can bring you the most revenue is a choice you must make if you are struggling to meet payroll.

If you are only concerned about the well-being of your patients and not the profitability of your practice, that is your choice.

But if your practice is not profitable, at some point you may not be able to stay in practice. And that is of no help to anyone.

Some patients (and the procedures you perform on those patients) are more profitable than others.

WHICH OF THESE CHALLENGES ARE HAPPENING IN YOUR PRACTICE?

Unlike other businesses, as a doctor or other health care provider, you have several unique challenges that cause tight cash flow... as well as some outright leaks. Even practices that are seen as highly successful can feel the strain of cash-flow problems.

Critical Cash Gaps can be triggered before and after a claim is filed when the following things happen in your practice:

- **Not enough patient appointments** to fill the daily schedule. This is a marketing problem.

- **Failure to check eligibility** prior to the office visit rather than prior to filing the claims.

- **Not discussing the financial obligation** with the patient before the office visit.

- **Failure to double check and update all patient information** prior to the visit and upon arrival. This can dramatically slow down reimbursements if there are errors. Also, verifying a match between the patient and the insurance card can catch usage by a family member who isn't covered. Ask for a picture ID for confirmation.

- **Inaccurate or incomplete superbill** or encounter form. Without correct diagnosis and treatment information, you won't get proper reimbursement.

- **Failure to make sure all patients check out** after the visit to settle co-payments. Patients can unknowingly walk out without paying, assuming insurance will cover the visit. Some *knowingly* walk out with their superbill or encounter form in hand, making billing impossible. In many cases you can also collect co-payments in advance for routine visits.

- **No-shows**. Few doctors charge for no-shows because of the fall-out of goodwill between the patient and doctor. Also, these bills are notoriously difficult to collect.

- **Lost patients** due to poor patient relations or inattention. Like every other business, a patient who stays with you yields more profit since you don't have any "new patient" expense attached to repeat visits.

- **Excessive write-offs**. The two reasons for write-offs are contractual adjustments and uncollectible accounts.

With an HMO or PPO, you may lose up to 36% on regular rates, depending on the agreement.

Uncollectible accounts from private-pay patients can run 5 to 15% among the affluent and up to 75% or more in lower-income patients.

Medicare write-offs vary by community, but about 35% is not unusual.

Competition can affect write-offs. Areas with widespread managed care tend to have more write-offs than communities with less managed care coverage.

This confirms that the way the health care system is currently structured doctors are almost guaranteed to experience cash-flow problems. The only issue is that it will be less or more – depending on your area of specialty, the community, and the proportion of payments due from patients, the government or private insurers.

Critical Cash Gaps lasting a few weeks to many months can occur between the date you provide the services and the date you finally get the check.

In addition, if you have to use a line of credit, for example, to cover expenses, the delayed payments are costing you money.

Blaming insurance companies, Medicare and Medicaid is easy to do. But practices also contribute to the problems. There are ways to speed up payments, collect more of what you're owed and plug the "internal bleeding" caused within your own office.

TYPICAL MISTAKES MADE WHEN YOU HAVE CASH-FLOW PROBLEMS

- Claims are not filed promptly.
- Patient information is not accurate or up to date.
- Claims are sent to the wrong place.
- Coding problems cause rejections.
- Properly prepared claims aren't paid for 30-120 days by insurance companies, Medicare or Medicaid.
- Patients owe balances for services not covered by insurance. You become the "bank" and must issue invoices and follow up.
- Patients can't or won't pay, causing write-offs.
- Collection agencies can be bad for patient relations and can cost upwards of 50% of the money collected.
- You have to borrow money to cover expenses while waiting for payments that may arrive in weeks, months... or never.

CHALLENGES YOU MAY NEED TO DEAL WITH

Some insurance companies refuse – or delay – paying what's rightfully due.

Other carriers have low reimbursements that require you to see more patients to net the same money.

If your expenses and payroll are out of control as well, you're putting additional pressure on the cash flow and may find yourself in a perpetual cash crunch.

You can put down your stethoscope and pick up a magnifying glass to play Sherlock. Have your office staff walk you through every point of patient contact from the initial phone call to a paid claim. You may discover that you've made assumptions about how things are being handled up front while you're busy in the back.

Look at every step through the cash-flow lens. You'll see how to plug many of the leaks in the pipeline that cost you money before and during the office visit (or surgery, treatment or consultation).

Include your back office in the review. Inventory control is crucial, as well as appropriately treating patients in the most efficient way. Then....

- **Let your staff help** you formulate improved systems and office procedures. The people on the front lines always know about problems the boss doesn't see.

- **Make employees aware** of the factors that stall cash flow. Let them know they have a stake in keeping the practice healthy and profitable.

- **Institute simple checklists** to make sure all the bases are covered. Make it known that these aren't recommendations, but the expected standard.

- **Document the procedures** you want implemented and review them with new and existing staff.

- **Monitor improvements monthly.** Reward the staff for actively improving cash flow and income by using the system... and by random acts of efficiency.

These suggestions are simple and obvious. Yet many medical offices simply muddle along in the same old way, blaming everything but their own actions for a cash crunch.

> *You're in a profession designed to create cash-flow problems. To get the most money into your practice - and the most out of it - you must go on the offensive.*

Fortunately, there are proven systems to handle the worst leaks in your practice, the ones stemming from medical claims and patients who owe you money.

- With the right billing partner you can slash rejected claims from a typical average of 30% to an enviable 2%.

- You can make sure you receive the patient's monthly payments on time for the balances they couldn't pay at the time the service was provided.

- You can collect on the old accounts receivable that you're about to write off without hiring a lawyer or using a collection agency.

THE PROBLEMS THAT PLAGUE MEDICAL BILLING

There are universal problems that doctors face when billing third parties for patient visits, treatments, or medical products and services. None of this will be news to you, but it's a real wake-up call when you see how the medical claims process can cause a major cash crunch in your practice. This should motivate you to make sure you're using the best system (or billing service) for your practice.

Many businesses can pinpoint a single glitch in a billing process to end a cash-flow problem. In contrast, doctors and other medical providers have many points in the process that can delay, reduce or prevent payment altogether. We touched on some of these in the last chapter, but now we're going to look at fixable problems that can plug leaks related to the filing of claims.

As you read the next few pages and relate them to various problems in your own practice, you may feel like you're picking your way through a mine field. However, identifying the extent of the problem will pave the way to eliminating medical claims as the biggest cash-flow killer in your practice.

Rejections have held steady at about 30% industry-wide. The smallest error can trigger a rejection. Every item must be perfect to be processed by the payer, whether it's Medicare or other insurers.

Keith Borglum, owner of Management & Marketing in Santa Rosa, California, tells of one medical practice that had a 71% error rate in a single year. This caused an estimated loss to the practice of $185,000.

COMMON CAUSES OF REJECTION

- **Billing for a procedure not covered.** As mentioned in the last chapter, this is an internal problem at the medical office that can be avoided by a staff member verifying coverage with a phone call *before* the patient arrives for an appointment.

- **Inaccurate coding.** This can be due to lack of knowledge on the part of the staff or poor communication from the doctor to ensure that the right code is used. Not keeping up with code changes is another likely cause of rejected claims.

- **Under-coding.** For many doctors, the fear of over-coding or unbundling results in employees being so cautious that the claim is actually miscoded.

- **Human error.** Typos, transposition of numbers and other mistakes in entry can cause a rejection.

- **Slow payments** – 30, 60, 90, 120 days or longer. The delays can be caused on the side of the practice or the side of the insurers responsible for payment.

- **Overwhelmed staff, slow submissions.** The quicker you can get accurate claims submitted, the faster you'll receive payment. You should know how long it takes for a claim to be filed.

- **Sluggish submissions by an outsourced medical biller.** If you use a medical biller, it's important to know how quickly the claims are being handled. If you're not asking for reports, you may not know when a given claim was submitted. The clock doesn't start for the insurer until the claim is received.

- **Ineffective rejected-claims management**. An inexperienced employee may not know how to resolve a particular problem with a claim. If it involves one or more calls to the insurer to resolve a legitimate claim, the value of that claim drops in proportion to the amount of time (money) it takes to get it paid.

- **Abandoned claims**. At some point, some claims can't be resolved by the person assigned to the job. It isn't at all uncommon for employees to finally give up and stuff these in a file in the bottom drawer.

  This is laughingly called the *Porsche Drawer* in some practices, because so much money is tied up in the claims.

WHY UNCOLLECTED CLAIMS SHOULD BE ON YOUR RADAR

Unresolved claims have a direct and immediate impact on cash flow. Every claim left to age without any attention is destined to be a write-off unless strong, effective action is taken.

This is lost money that has cost you more than you may realize:

First, you provided the service.

Second, you paid to have the claim filed.

Third, you repeatedly paid to sort out the problem that prevented payment.

Finally, you've had to cover expenses with money from sources other than the payments you were expecting from these claims. You may have even paid to borrow money.

Uncollected claims may reflect poorly on the employees. If you scrutinize rejected claims, you may find that the source of the problem wasn't actually an uncooperative insurance company or lack of help at Medicare (although those are easy default targets that are rarely challenged).

If employees know that they, or their office-mates, were sloppy in the first place, they may want to bury the problem. Strict reporting systems can make it harder to cover up internal procedural errors that are costing you money.

Any unpaid claims that are essentially uncollectible are skewing your actual financial picture. When a sizable chunk of your money is either uncollected or uncollectible, any cash-flow projections you make that include accounts receivable are flawed.

You may find yourself in a cash crunch without warning, simply because the abandoned claims became "phantom cash" without your knowledge.

Unpaid bills that aren't reflected in the books are also distorting your actual financial position. This can happen because the staff gets behind. It can also occur when employees simply don't understand the importance of accurate accounts payable lists. You can't project cash flow if you don't know what's been paid and what's outstanding.

Employees may not think it matters that much. If the attitude you project is that uncollected claims are annoying, but unavoidable, the employees will assume the same posture.

Instead, assume an attitude of relentless pursuit of what is owed to the practice. Show the employees how payments affect them, their income, and even any extras you can give them, not just your ability to pay for a new luxury car. Consider bonuses or perks based on improvements.

Medical software. The introduction of medical software was an enormous leap for doctors previously forced to fill out forms by hand. There are a number of popular medical software packages, but software has built-in limitations.

Medical billing software is not cheap, but the initial price is not the only concern. Upgrades are costly and can run up to several thousands of dollars, depending on the company and the number of doctors in your practice. Even so, it's the option many medical practices choose.

Changes in CPT and ICD Codes and the Health Insurance Portability and Accountability Act may be in effect before an upgrade is offered by your software company... and even longer if you delay in buying and installing your upgrade. This opens the door for rejected claims due to miscoding and problems due to non-compliance with HIPAA regulations.

If you outsource your medical billing, you may not know what software is being used. You also may not know if they're upgrading in a timely way… or at all. Outsourcing is an economical choice, but only if your billing service is up to date so you're always compliant.

Some small medical billers may find the high price of upgrades out of reach. If you currently outsource to a billing service using software, be sure to ask whether they're current with all system and coding updates. Otherwise, you're risking rejection of claims and HIPAA compliance issues.

Software can have unexpected technical issues. If a young assistant is typing information into the software and there's a glitch, tech support is typically available quickly if you've bought from a reputable software company.

The question is not whether tech support is available, it's how long it will take to resolve any problems. And does your data entry person have more than keyboard skills so she can implement what the support technician tells her to do?

By the time the problem is fixed, there may be a backlog of claims to file, which in turn delays payment. That's how a technical problem can turn into a cash-flow problem.

SERVER-BASED SOFTWARE VS. CLOUD-BASED BILLING SYSTEMS

Let's clarify what "electronic billing" means in relation to the government mandate.

Many doctors assume that working with software is, by definition, "electronic billing." There are many people - both in medical offices and medical billing services - who've generated their claims with software, then printed them out and put them in the mail.

More recently, software users would generate the claims using software and then upload batches to a clearinghouse or payer.

Technically speaking, software does drive cloud-based systems, so there remains some confusion about the use of the term "software."

For our purposes, "software" means a billing program that resides on a computer in a doctor's office or at a medical billing service.

True electronic billing is *completing* and *submitting claims online*, not just preparing the claim by computer using software installed on the hard drive before uploading it in batches to a clearinghouse.

That means that your current medical biller - either in-house or outsourced - has to submit the claims to a clearinghouse electronically. This creates a two-step process: generate the claims; submit the claims in batches.

1. **The software/submit process.** has three main points, depending on the features available on the software used, that often sabotage timely payments.

2. **Checking for accuracy manually.** Some strides have been made to give the individual entering the data some assurance that the claims don't have glaring flaws in the document that would trigger a rejection. However, the burden of inputting correct numbers ultimately rests with the human operator. Certain coding errors, for example, may not be caught prior to submission of a claim.

3. **Batches are checked by the payer for problems.** As mentioned earlier, the sooner you can notice the smallest discrepancy of information, the sooner you can get paid. Any delay causes the batch to be kicked back. In submitting, that means the person may have to start collecting from the day the error was present, tracking down and fixing errors in a batch of claims. This is lost time for the biller and likely more expense for the medical practice.

In contrast, a cloud-based solution eliminates these and other problems for you automatically.

When evaluating a cloud-based, electronic claims filing system or outsourced service, make sure it meets the current state-of-the-art criteria:

1. **Claims are completed online.** It's a seamless process to generate a claim and submit it.

2. **Automatic real-time checking.** If there's a coding discrepancy or some other questionable entry, the system automatically flags the potential problem and won't allow the person to proceed until the issue is resolved.

3. **Code and HIPAA updates are made as they occur.** The correct information is available the next time the online system is accessed.

However, software on a computer must be updated by installing the latest upgrade. Some practices, or their billers, delay getting new upgrades due to the expense. Others want to avoid the hassle and downtime required to install the current software.

Coding errors account for many rejections. Being current is one of the keys to higher accuracy.

- There are no upgrade charges - ever - when codes or HIPAA changes are made in a cloud-based system. This can save hundreds or thousands of dollars a year, depending on the size of the practice. Changes are made as they are issued at no additional charge. (If you outsource to a medical biller using the system, they won't have any extra expense for upgrades, which helps to keep costs down for you.)

The most compelling reason to utilize state-of-the-art electronic claims filing is because...

- The ideal system can reduce claim rejections from the industry average of approximately 30% down to less than 2%.

- Claims are typically paid in as few as seven days, with an average of 14 days from submission to payment.

If there were no other advantages to using web-based, real-time filing, getting 98% of your claims through the first time and receiving payments within days instead of months are reasons enough. That will have a major positive impact on your cash flow.

If you have a small practice, you may think this has nothing to do with you. But it does.

ADVANTAGES OF CLOUD-BASED BILLING SYSTEMS

Computer-based software just can't match the efficiency and economy of real-time, cloud-based filing. Doctors expect technology to improve diagnosis and treatment. In the same way, they expect technology to serve their practices. Since there are clear advantages, and no downside, the sooner you move to a web-based system, the faster you'll see bottom-line results.

In the meantime, get your cash flow moving by switching now or finding a billing company that utilizes a cloud-based system. The promise of this chapter is to put more money in your pocket faster. Cloud-based electronic billing is the only certain way to accomplish this… quickly.

THE CASE FOR OUTSOURCING YOUR BILLING NOW

If you're currently handling your claims in-house, it may be time to look at outsourcing to save money, stress and needless activity in your office. Many practices seem to be more absorbed in paperwork and billing activities than they are with the patients.

There are often as many administrative employees as health care professionals (or more). Is this really how you want to run your practice? By outsourcing, the costs related to filing claims are also lower than having your own staff complete and submit them.

The New England Journal of Medicine reported that the administrative costs and related expenses comprise 26.9% of the physician's gross income. This equals about 1.5 employees per doctor at an average salary of $51,564 per employee, not including benefits such as vacation.

David Jakielo detailed the advantages of outsourcing in his article "Why Doctors Should Outsource Their Billing" in *BC Advantage Magazine*. He cited the complexity of medical billing compared to a few years ago. Rejections were around 5%. Now he tells his clients:

> *"Never do anything that you can have someone else do more efficiently and at a lesser cost."*

For medical bills, using an online system can be extremely efficient and pass the savings along to you. Pricing depends, of course, on the complexity of the claims. Fees can be as low as 5-8% of the claim. The medical billing service typically doesn't get paid for a claim until it's paid, so outsourcing does not contribute to a cash crunch.

One question that many doctors ask is, "How can I be sure that outsourcing my billing will reduce my claims filing costs?"

As with all services you outsource, you'll want to be able to have an apples-to-apples comparison of what you're paying now and what you'll save with a service utilizing a cloud-based billing system. At the very least, you want to make sure you won't be paying more.

Whatever outsourced services you consider should be able to produce a side-by-side comparison to show you how they can save you money.

From a cash-smart standpoint, we believe that outsourcing is more cost-effective than hiring employees to do the work. Even so, some doctors simply want to have the control of claims in their own offices.

If you choose this option for your web-based solution, make sure you can get technical support and training for your staff. Depending on the system, almost anyone who can type can enter the data. However, you still want to have someone to call for questions or for training a new employee on the system.

It's also prudent to make sure experienced coding specialists are available to your staff. Although most online systems are simple enough for almost anyone to use and check for correct codes, some cases may require seldom-used or unfamiliar codes that must be clarified.

Savings and convenience make a strong argument for outsourcing the entire operation. And here's another...

CLOUD-BASED CLAIMS FILING IS MORE SECURE

Some doctors, maybe you, believe that confidential patient information is safe if all the information is stored on computers in the office.

On the face of it, that makes sense. But in reality, you are no less vulnerable to theft than any other business. You may have files meticulously backed up, but if a computer is stolen, that information is at risk.

Perhaps you use a computer-based medical billing service. The security of your data depends on your vendor's ability to keep the computer safe.

WARNING: Software installed on a local computer containing all your patient data, at either a medical billing service or your own office, is vulnerable to hardware "crashes" and theft. This also exposes you to non-compliance with HIPAA rules and regulations, for which you can be fined.

CLOUD-BASED CLAIMS FILING SYSTEMS SOLVES THESE CONCERNS

- All the claims are completed on a secure, encrypted site. No files are kept on your local hard drive.

- Routine, secure backup. All the information is on a password-protected area secured for your patient and claims data only. Multiple backup sites across North America make the system disaster-proof. Hard copies are available if you need them.

- Security meets or exceeds the hacker-proof standards used by financial institutions, Internet banking, credit card companies, online stock trading companies and government agencies.

- HIPAA compliant. If concerns about HIPAA compliance have kept you trapped by paper bills, or you're not sure your current medical biller is up to date, web-based filing can put your mind at ease.

- Password-protected access. Your data is accessible only to those with a password.

- Access information from any computer online. The data is encrypted, so you or your staff can have access to your patient information at any time, 24/7. You can see exactly what's going on with a particular claim, and your billing service is more accountable because you know precisely when a claim was filed. There are no blind spots. The system is transparent.

- A number of reports let you stay on top of outstanding claims. When you firmly understand the cash-flow impact of your claims, you'll appreciate having a choice of financial reports such as day sheets, patient or insurance aging reports, and financial summaries. All your information is available to you 24/7 from any computer with Internet access.

- Posting payments is easy and fast. This keeps you up to date on money flowing into the practice.

CLAIMS CAN BE YOUR BIGGEST LEAK IN YOUR CASH-FLOW

If your practice is growing, it's unlikely that claims filing will get any easier using less efficient systems.

If your current system isn't getting claims filed as quickly as possible, or you wait longer than 30 days to get paid for most of your claims, you have a chronic cash-flow problem. It won't go away until you switch to cloud-based, real-time electronic billing or outsource your billing to a company that uses the latest cloud-based system.

WHY YOU MUST COLLECT PATIENT RECEIVABLES

If a friend told you she was going to open a retail store, knowing ahead of time that she'd collect less than half of the money she billed to customers, what would you tell her? Right. "You can't make it if you let you customers give themselves a 50% discount on their purchases."

That is no less true for you as a doctor, but that is the nationwide average of patient receivables that are never collected.

But you do have options. You don't have to sacrifice good business practice for the sake of patients.

We're about to show you a better way… one that will keep your cash flowing… even if you have to allow monthly payments.

But first, let's look at why the problem of patient payments is so entrenched in the medical industry.

A portion of almost every practice's income is directly tied to payments by patients… and their ability to pay. As a doctor, you already know the reasons that contribute to hefty accounts receivable from your patients:

- Co-payments of 15-25%, depending on the insurance plan of the patient.
- Services that aren't covered by insurance.

Uninsured patients who must pay their own medical bills. According to CoverTheUninsured.org, more than 47 million Americans are uninsured.

With more businesses eliminating health insurance as a benefit, these figures will continue to rise.

Underinsured patients may have limited coverage to conserve on insurance premiums, which leaves them liable for the cost of certain medical services.

> *Doctors commonly just accept that they have to bear the burden of extending credit. However, to move from cash crunch to cash flow, you must be willing to retool your system to prevent inevitable cash-flow problems caused by slow- and no-pay patients.*

Slow or no payment often starts with poor payment policies or the casual attitude of the practice toward collecting money. Late payments or no payments create Critical Cash Gaps.

WHAT TO DO WHEN PATIENT PAYMENTS ARE DELAYED

Patients are unaware of how much they will have to pay. As mentioned before, this can be covered in the pre-visit conversation.

If the doctor decides to do an unscheduled procedure on the spot - either because it's prudent to do so or just "so you don't have to come back a second time" - the patient should be told the amount they will have to pay. A patient may not have come prepared to pay for more than a simple office visit and should be given the option to postpone the procedure.

Charges that should be covered by insurance roll over to the patient in error. By policy, most doctors hold the patients responsible for any charges that aren't covered by insurance.

However, when claims are rejected, some offices aren't careful to confirm the real source of the problem, which can be fixed. The practice then burdens the patients with fees they can't afford, and you never get paid.

For example, one obstetrical practice discovered that claims were being rejected because new babies had not been properly enrolled in the insurance program by the parents. By waiting until the newborn was enrolled to submit claims, the doctors were paid.

There's no clear patient payment policy. A sign on the wall that "payment is due at the time of service" is a wake-up call or a reminder. But that's not the same as a written policy, complete with the options you offer.

For example, some practices don't accept American Express. If that's the card the patient planned to use, they may not have a back-up option in hand when they check out.

You're too willing to be the "bank" for patients. Some practices don't press for full payment of the patient's amount due and offer to bill for the rest automatically.

Many don't charge interest, even when they carry balances for extended periods of time. This sparks additional problems...

You become a low-cost HMO by default. Putting patients on minimum monthly payments and not adjusting the amounts for subsequent visits - which result in higher balances owed - is great for your patients, but disastrous for your cash flow.

You allow 60-90 days to elapse on a bill that remains unpaid - or is only partially paid - before suggesting a structured payment plan. Furniture or appliance stores may sell with a "90 days like cash" offer, but their profit margins often allow for such financing. Yours don't.

You're passive about collections. You and your staff are shy about reminding Mrs. Smith she's overdue. Bless her heart, she does the best she can. And the Fosters have five children and can hardly manage.

In an effort to not offend, or be seen as anything but the hero, you may be making it easy for patients to shuffle your invoices to the side again and maybe catch up next month.

It costs more to collect than the balance that's due. According to one study, costs per paper invoice are now up to more than $34 with all factors considered (labor, materials, postage, etc.). If you have to send multiple bills to collect, the value of the amount due is diminished.

Okay. So billing patients is a mess, no matter how you look at it. But of greater concern is, why won't they pay? Is it simply lack of funds? Or is something else going on?

THINGS THAT CONTRIBUTE TO SLOW OR NO PAYMENTS

And yes, not having enough money is one of them. Some families are truly on the edge, including two-income families who would be considered financially stable or even affluent.

The foreclosure of large numbers of McMansions in cities across the country is a visible signal that the appearance of affluence may be based on overextended credit and risky financial practices.

It's also a matter of priorities. Human nature being what it is, especially in America, people have short attention spans. And our priorities shift with the seasons.

For example, if you're billing families just prior to the opening of school, their available cash may be going to clothes and school supplies. Through the holidays and after, with December bills arriving in the new year, your bill can settle at the bottom of the pile.

Most people don't intend on stiffing you for the money they owe you. But really, what leverage do you have?

Not paying you doesn't mean they aren't able to get other things they really want - from basics like power and phone service to discretionary expenses such as cable, a new car or a vacation. Mrs. Smith is planning to take a cruise and the Fosters just got a new ATV.

If you don't get paid, there's nothing to take back.

Of course, if you're working with patients who are over their heads in heavy debts because of payments for an extended illness, you'll handle those on a case-by-case basis. What we're talking about here are your mainstream patients.

PLUG CRITICAL CASH GAPS WITH THESE PATIENT-FRIENDLY POLICIES

Your first line of defense is to make it clear that you're serious about having payments made in full when services are delivered.

Have your payment policy on the clipboard, ready for a signature, along with the other forms new patients fill out. Mail out your new policy to existing patients and remind them when they come to the office.

Think about it. Your ability to deliver quality care is based on being able to be paid appropriately - and on time - for your services.

First, make it clear you expect full payment...

- Cash. Some practices have to scramble to accept cash if they commonly receive payments by check or credit card. Keep plenty of change on hand and institute a cash check-out system.

- Checks. Be sure you use all the precautions available to prevent bad checks. Laws vary by state.

- Debit cards. The use of debit cards is most widespread among those under 30. More than half of American consumers are using their debit card instead of checks when making purchases.

- Credit cards. Used almost universally, credit cards shift the risk from your practice to the credit card company. In your written policy, specify the cards you accept so there's no confusion and there are no awkward moments (and no lost payment) when a patient presents a card you don't accept.

OTHER OPTIONS WHEN THE PATIENT CAN'T PAY IN FULL

Here's your challenge: You must make a clear distinction between the people who don't want to pay in full and those who can't pay in full.

Well-to-do patients may assume their business is valuable to you and that you're eager to have them as patients. They make large purchases at clothing stores and other retailers and expect to be billed.

And while you want to have a patient-friendly environment in your practice, allowing or even encouraging this type of behavior is a quick step closer to a Critical Cash Gap.

Your affluent patients may request more extensive services and be willing to pay for them. But if you carry their payments, that's a bad deal for you.

In contrast, those with financial challenges may have a sense that you're required to extend credit terms. This simply isn't true. However, based on your current demographic profile, it may be obvious that you must have a back-up plan readily available for a segment of your patients.

Some cloud-based practice management systems have a "portal" that the patient can log into and set up automated payments or just make individual payments when they wish.

HERE ARE THREE PATIENT PAYMENT SOLUTIONS

1. **Automatic credit card payments.** This option allows you to bill credit cards monthly in manageable amounts that both you and the patient negotiate.

   Pros: You get paid without having to send out any bills or dunning reminders.

   Cons: This can become an administrative nightmare that can result in payments never being billed if there is no automatic system in place. You'll need an Internet-based "virtual terminal" to set up these automated payments, or find a billing service that can handle monthly billing for you.

Current credit card interest rates (excluding short-term, low-interest promotional rates) range from 7.9% to 25.24%.[4]

Patients know that if they miss a payment, they may trigger penalty rates which are, on average, 24.51% and as high as 32.24%. Consumer Action's 2007 Credit Card Survey reported that 85% of credit card companies now enforce penalty rates. This fact alone may keep some patients from using this option, but they'll also be reluctant if they know they're very close to their credit limit and want to keep what credit they have open for living expenses.

The downside for you is that it costs you to offer this option. As a doctor, you're still a "merchant" to the credit card company and you pay both a transaction fee and a percentage of the amount charged.

Fees have several components, including the interchange rate, discount rate, transaction fee and any other charges related to providing the service.

Most doctors want to offer credit card acceptance to those patients who prefer to use them and have adequate lines of credit. You owe it to yourself to make sure you're getting the lowest effective rate.

2. **Third-party lenders specializing in medical loans.** You've probably been approached to offer - or are currently offering - these types of loans.

   Pros: You can transfer the full risk of the bill to a financial institution and get your money.

   Cons: Like other loans, a patient has to be credit-worthy to qualify. In some cases, the loans require home ownership and are essentially home equity loans. That means some people can't qualify and others don't want to risk their homes.

3. **Pre-authorized payments.** This plan allows patients to make payments using automated monthly withdrawals from their bank accounts. This eliminates your monthly invoicing and collection problems.

This third option is the simplest way to quickly resolve your patient payment problem. Some systems and patient portals allow patients to manage their payments online.

WHY YOU SHOULD SCRUTINIZE ALL EXPENSES

Take a look at each expense and ask:

- What is this for?
- Do I need it?
- Can I reduce or eliminate it?
- Can I get a better price somewhere else?

Make sure that all of the expenses make sense. Employees can commit theft by creating shell businesses and sending payments to themselves.

Here are a few examples of ways you can plug spending leaks:

- Sub-lease unused office space
- Find a new vendor for supplies
- Take advantage of sales

Look into partnering with other practices to share resources like a copier or make large purchases at a lower unit price. Consider a captive medical malpractice insurance plan. Claim all tax deductions.

HOW TO PROTECT AGAINST THEFT, FRAUD AND EMBEZZLEMENT

Medical practices have the highest embezzlement rate of any service industry. According to an MGMA study, 83% of medical practices report that they have been victims of embezzlement.

Here are some steps you can take to decrease the risk of theft at your office.

Hire the right people. Verify the information provided by the applicant. Call references. Conduct a criminal and credit check for all new employees.

Develop policies, procedures and protocols. Create a written policy outlining your zero tolerance of fraud, and have each employee sign it.

Nearly half of all theft involves cash from co-pays or petty cash. Do what you can to keep honest people honest.

- Use a lockbox for petty cash.
- Divide financial duties. The person collecting the cash should be different than the person reconciling transactions.

Implement safe banking practices

- Restrict signature authority of checks
- Get rid of signature stamps
- Restrict online banking access
- Pay bills online
- Get bank statements sent to your home

Purchase business liability insurance that includes coverage for employee theft and embezzlement. Bond all staff who process payments.

Know the warning signs. Worrisome employee behavior includes:

- Spending habits that exceed salaries
- Refusal to take vacations or time off
- Unusual or long work hours
- Taking accounting books home
- Missing receipts, invoices or purchase orders
- Overdue notices from vendors
- Patient complaints about billing errors
- Unexplained shortages of petty cash
- Unusual patterns in bank deposit statements

Listen to your gut. If you are worried about an employee, don't dismiss the concern.

SUMMARY

- Your time is valuable. Every activity in your practice takes time away from other activities. Decide which activities could be eliminated and which should take more of your time.

- Cash-flow determines whether you can stay in private practice or not. You must take time each week to make sure you are getting paid for all the activities you and your staff perform.

- You (and your staff) were trained to provide medical services to patients, not bookkeeping functions. There are companies who deal with the billing functions for physicians on a daily basis and who keep up with the changes in insurance and government rules and regulations. Let them do their job while you focus on yours.

ACTION STEPS:

✓ Identify and focus on profitable activities in your practice.

✓ Locate the leaks in your cash flow and scrutinize all expenses.

✓ Consider focusing on your core competency and outsource your billing.

8

LET'S TALK ABOUT WEALTH

I t's not what you make; it's what you keep.

How do you translate your revenue into wealth? This is quite literally the million-dollar question.

What is wealth?

Wealth is a state of prosperity that gives you the freedom to do what you want to do when you want to do it.

Vicki's investments gave her the safety net to leave her conventional surgical practice and launch into a career as an author, speaker and consultant.

> *Wealth gives you the freedom to choose how long you continue to practice medicine.*

A doctor in his 80s may go to work every day because it still brings him delight.

Unfortunately, half of physicians are behind where they would like to be in retirement planning. They look ahead and see that they will NEED to work to pay their bills.

What is the Difference Between Revenue and Wealth?

Your practice's revenue represents your compensation for the services you offer. You work for this money.

As you accumulate assets, you can put your money to work for you. Most physicians have the goal of replacing their practice income with investment income in retirement.

How does a physician - or anyone else - build wealth?

The financial prescription for building wealth is simple:

- Spend less than you earn.

- Start saving early. Einstein calls compound interest the eighth wonder of the world.

- Marry the right person. (So says Vicki's mentor Dr. John Ryan.)

- Protect what you have.

Wealth-building is a balancing act. How much will you defer pleasure today to enjoy financial freedom tomorrow?

Are You Anywhere Near Ready for Retirement?

The evolving fields of behavioral finance and neuro-economics attempt to explain investors' observed behaviors. Here are a few highlights:

- Investors behave irrationally, making predictable mistakes.

- We have an aversion to loss, and tend to take high risk to protect against losses.

- We may have a biologic set-point that determines an individual's propensity to spend or save.

- We ascribe relative value to resources. Give a monkey an apple and he is happy. Give another monkey two apples and take away one, and he is angry. Both monkeys have the same resources.

In other words, investors act like your patients! Compliance is a huge issue.

Physicians as a group are wealthy, right?

Wrong!

Physicians earn top dollars. The U.S. Bureau of Labor Statistics culled data from tax records to conclude that nine of the top ten earners in the U.S. call themselves a "doctor."

In a recent survey, half of all physicians are behind where they would like to be in retirement planning. Professional medical associations are exploring how to access competency in older physicians who continue to practice because they cannot afford to retire.

Why Do Physicians Have a Hard Time Building Wealth?

Here are some unique financial challenges that physicians face:

- Medical school debt
- A late start on earning and savings
- The potential loss of assets from known and overlooked risks
- A high tax burden
- A propensity to get investment advice from the wrong people
- Vulnerability to fraud and theft

One of the greatest threats to a physician's wealth is the DDD - dumb doctor deal. Many physicians turn to colleagues for investing advice. A physician's excellent clinical judgment does not uniformly translate to excellent investing judgment.

Five Most Common Financial Mistakes Physicians Make?

Here are 5 common financial mistakes physicians make, and strategies to avoid them.

Mistake #1: Imbalance between spending and savings.

For an investor time works like gravity. An early start on savings is like riding a bike downhill; conversely, a late start means pedaling uphill.

We physicians already get a late start on saving because of our prolonged training period and the burden of medical school debt. After all the years of deprivation, many physicians feel it's time to live it up once training is over. It's easy to grow into and spend any level of income.

The evolving field of neuro-economics suggests that biology may play a role in an individual's propensity to save or spend. Some people are born "spenders" and others are born "savers."

While biology is not destiny, it takes self-discipline for spenders to save - and for savers to spend. Discipline is like a muscle, and gets fatigued with prolonged use.

Here are some ways to save more:

- **Automate savings**. If you don't see the money, you will not miss it as much!

- As you anticipate a financial windfall - whether it's an inheritance, the transition from training to a career launch or a higher salary in a new position - **plan to save a high percentage of the increase.**

- **Form a clear multi-sensory picture of your desired future.** It's easier to say no to something today when there's a picture of a brighter tomorrow.

Mistake #2: Getting financial advice from the wrong people.

Many physicians turn to their colleagues for financial advice. Vicki thinks of all the investment opportunities she heard about in the surgeon's lounge. Most physicians who jumped into these schemes lost their money.

One financial advisor says that one of her major jobs is protecting her doctor clients from those dumb doctor deals.

Here are steps you can take:

- Ask yourself, "Do I really trust the person who is giving me advice?"

- Ask your colleagues, "Who helps you plan for retirement? What do you like about working with this person?" Hopefully your physician clients say nice things about you!

- Ask yourself, "How will I objectively evaluate investing opportunities?"

Mistake #3: Failing to manage taxes wisely.

Proactive tax management correlates with the ability to build wealth.

You also know that CPAs work hard to ensure that clients minimize their tax burdens in any given year.

You see the bigger picture. You know that taxes will go up, and that contributions to a tax-deferred retirement account will, in fact, be taxed. Find and work with a team of consultants who see the big tax picture for both today and tomorrow.

Mistake #4: Failing to protect assets.

You carry insurance on your homes and cars. You have a medical malpractice policy. You may even insure your smartphone.

Still, many physicians do not insure their most valuable asset: their ability to generate income.

Furthermore, they may not see how the activities of their partners impact their ability to build wealth. When a life partner over-spends, or a business partner commits Medicare fraud, the physician can pay the price.

Here are steps you can take:

- Ask yourself, "Am I prepared for the "what if's" in life?" In addition to life and disability insurance, look into an umbrella policy for your home. Check with your medical malpractice carrier and see if you are protected for claims arising from social media activity.

- Talk with your client about incorporating - even if they are employed. Ask, "Can you trust your colleagues to do the right thing?"

- Ask yourself, "Do you and your life partner have an agreement about how to manage money that works for both of you? Are you raising financially literate children?

Mistake #5: Ignoring the human condition.

Nobel laureate Daniel Kahneman studied how people respond to changing markets including the 2002 dot-com bust and real estate boom. He concludes that investors make irrational choices.

Predictable investing errors are part of the human condition.

If you have ever looked at optical illusions, you know how easy it is to fool the brain. Yet, even after someone proves that we have been tricked, our false perceptions persist.

Here are some of the predictable errors that get in the way of building wealth; you see them every day.

- **Loss aversion.** We will take greater risks to avoid loss than to experience gains. That means investors take risks at the time they should be erring on the side of safety.

- **Over and under reactions.** Investors tend to behave with optimism when the market goes up, and become much more pessimistic when the market goes down.

- **Overconfidence.** Investors tend to overestimate their ability to beat the market, and underestimate investing challenges.

- **Relativity.** Investors see the world through the eyes of relative experience. Imagine how you would feel if someone gave you a gift card. Now imagine how you would respond if someone gave you two gift cards and took one back. You have the identical outcome in each case, but it feels much different.

- **Spending as a stress management tool.** Spending creates a positive feeling state through the release of dopamine. The medial pre-frontal cortex of the brain modulates this response. This part of the brain also regulates stress response. Could the growing numbers of physicians on the edge of burnout be spending as a stress management tool? An estimated 5 to 10% of Americans - including physicians - suffer from a shopping or gambling addiction.

Here are steps you can take:

- Observe your investing behaviors. When do you fall into these predictable traps, and how can you avoid them?

- Consider whether you are using spending as a stress management tool. Could you think of other healthier options?

- If you have concerns about possible shopping or gambling addictions, seek help. You are not alone.

ALL YOU NEED TO KNOW ABOUT ESTATE PLANNING

Work with a professional estate planner to ensure that the wealth you build will go to your heirs. This person can help you with your will and advanced directives.

What about retiring on the money you get from the sale of your practice?

Before you decide to fund your retirement with the sale of your practice, get more information. Consult with a professional who does practice valuation. Start optimizing the practice's value TODAY. It may be that an investment in social media, for example, could make a difference to the sale price.

Diversification - not putting all your eggs in one basket - is the safest way to approach retirement planning. The sale of your practice is potentially one source of revenue; talk with your financial advisor about others.

How do you decide how to allocate your income? How do you balance paying your medical school debt and planning for your kids' education? How much should you be investing and saving? How much house do you really want to buy? An experienced financial advisor can help you make sense of these questions.

HOW DO YOU EVALUATE INVESTMENT OPPORTUNITIES?

Many investment opportunities will come your way. Should you purchase your practice building? Invest in oil wells? Buy rental properties? What about a vacation home?

Again, your financial advisor can help you vet investment opportunities and protect you from those pesky dumb doctor deals.

WORK WITH A PROFESSIONAL FINANCIAL ADVISOR?

While the basic wealth-building concepts are simple, there are many moving parts. You balance today's financial needs with your retirement goals.

Today, half of physicians work with professional financial advisors; the other half are financial do-it-yourselfers. The physicians who work with professional financial advisors are more secure in their retirement preparedness.

If you have gotten through medical school, you can master finances. You can also mow your own lawn, do your own cleaning or prepare your own taxes.

The question is whether you want to invest your time and energy into learning about how to build wealth. Doing the things you do well and delegating all other tasks is usually the wisest choice.

HOW DO YOU FIND A GOOD FINANCIAL ADVISOR, CPA OR ESTATE PLANNER?

Ask your colleagues for referrals. You want to work with professionals who work with physicians like you every day.

Each professional, whether an estate planner, a tax attorney of financial advisor, has a different way of getting compensated. Your financial advisor may charge you a flat fee, or a percentage of assets under management.

The real question is not what you spend on your consultants; it's the return on your investment. You have millions of dollars on the line. This is not the time or place to pinch pennies; the stakes are too high. Get top-drawer advisors. The professional fees represent money well spent.

SUMMARY

- Wealth is the freedom to do what you want to do when you want to do it.

- Physicians and other investors make predictable financial mistakes that can be avoided.

- Gather a team that can help you build wealth.

ACTION STEPS:

- ✓ Define your financial goals.
- ✓ Identify your retirement plan.
- ✓ Assemble your wealth-building team.

9

GROOM LEADERS

> *"Leadership is communicating to people their worth and potential so clearly that they are inspired to see it in themselves."*
>
> —*Stephen Covey*

You are most likely reading this book because you see the need to make a change. How do you make the changes you envision and inspire those around you to get on board? This is where leadership comes into play.

WHAT IS LEADERSHIP?

Leaders are change agents. A leader helps others see a vision and translate a dream into reality. **In other words, leaders inspire people - themselves included - to conduct themselves differently.**

You serve as the leader of your medical team, your consultants and your staff. Your patients and perhaps their family members turn to you for leadership. You exercise self-leadership.

The problem is that we physicians are not formally taught leadership skills. Learning to lead is the old "see one, do one, teach one." We tend to imitate our mentors.

How Leadership Can Explode Your Practice's Growth

Improve patient compliance. When you inspire patients to take medication as prescribed, or implement the recommended lifestyle choices, you get better medical outcomes. This enhances your ability to get more referrals from more physicians, generate more revenue in a pay-for-performance world, and enhance your reputation in the medical community.

Improve the patient experience. All of your staff members represent your "brand." One negative experience can sour things and stand in the way of your practice's growth. Your ability to articulate your vision of the patients' experience to your staff and set behavioral expectations will promote growth.

Increase the numbers of referrals from physicians. Right now physicians have referral habits. How will you disrupt those habits and persuade them to try you? The status quo is a formidable foe.

Increase the numbers of referrals from patients. Your single best marketing tool is a delighted patient who tells others about you.

Avoid problems created by disruptive staff. Vicki recently spoke with a surgeon concerned about his rapidly falling fees. She asked him about his most pressing concern. He said, "My top concern is my junior colleague. He brings in lots of cases and gets good outcomes, but none of my staff want to work with him." Offering strong leadership helps avoid the problem of disruptive staff. Furthermore, offering self-leadership skills will decrease the incidence of disruptive behavior.

How Do You Inspire Others to Change?

Supporting behavioral changes is one of the most difficult tasks to accomplish. Think about your own life. Are you using the same toothpaste that you used as a child?

Do you take the exact same route to the office every day? Do you have a morning ritual?

Think about the last time you made a small change in your life. How easy or difficult was it for you to implement your new electronic medical record, or even a software update on your personal computer?

Now consider this question: when was the last time that you made a proactive, meaningful change in your life? It could be spending more time with your family, listening more or changing your eating habits.

The truth is that it is very difficult to change. Most New Year's resolutions are abandoned by late January.

Moreover, change is all but impossible unless and until the individual wants to change.

Simply put, you cannot "make" people change. However, you can identify the people who are open to change, create a vision and help them create an environment in which it's easier to make better choices.

POWERFUL PERSUASION TOOLS

You have three basic tools to persuade others to act in the ways you want. These are the same tools you use whether you're trying to get patients to take their medication as prescribed, get your daughter to practice the piano, or get more physicians to send you more patients.

1. **Persuasion through authority**

    The words, "Because I said so," had meaning in the Father-Knows-Best era. Mandates generally build walls between people instead of bridges. Effective practice-building is bridge-building, so this tactic is likely to drive people away from you instead of toward you.

    The mandate may be a law. For example, Washington State has imposed a legal mandate that requires physicians to make a pain clinic referral when patients exceed a set ceiling of opioid doses.

2. **Persuasion through logic and reason.**

    You can persuade through logic and reason. Here are some logical reasons physicians might refer patients to you:

You have unique access to resources. A primary care doctor cannot replace a mitral valve; only heart surgeons have privileges to do this procedure.

You use resources more effectively. Your experience translates to treatments with less time, less pain and/or less expense.

You get better results. Practice makes perfect.

Your campaign to influence those around you may include logic-based sharing of facts and figures about your training, your experience and your outcomes.

3. **Persuasion through emotion**

Neuroscience suggests that we make most of our choices with our limbic system (feeling brain) and justify them with our cerebral cortex (thinking brain). In other words, **emotion drives motion.**

Consider the possibility that most behaviors and choices are driven by emotion. You are most influential when you help another person achieve their desired emotional state. This is the driving force behind most of our actions.

What do people want? They want to be seen, heard and valued. They want to know, "Somebody understands me."

You are in the best position to persuade when the thing that's important to the other person becomes important to you.

> *"You can have everything in life you want, if you will just help enough other people get what they want."*
>
> *– Zig Ziglar*

HOW TO USE EMOTIONAL FORCES TO DRIVE HUMAN BEHAVIOR

You are most influential when you help another person achieve their desired emotional state.

Each of us has a temperamental affinity towards one of four emotional states: to be in control, to belong, to be admired or to be right. This affinity forms the basis of four personality types:

"**The Director**" thrives when getting results, wilts when losing control and likes feeling powerful. This is a common personality type for physicians.

"**The Team Player**" thrives when fitting in, wilts when standing out and likes a sense of belonging. This is a common personality type for nurses.

"**The Accountant**" thrives on being right, wilts when wrong and likes feeling smart. This personality type responds to your outcomes data and logical arguments.

"**The Actor**" thrives on admiration, wilts with disapproval and likes feeling important.

These emotional factors can either slow or accelerate appropriate referrals. The Director, for example, may see a referral as an admission of defeat. You overcome his resistance by reminding him how much more he would like to free up his time to see more of his best-fit patients.

FACTORS THAT ERODE YOUR ABILITY TO PERSUADE

Here are some factors that erode your ability to be a change agent.

The "**Eat your vegetables; they're good for you**" effect. We have a human aversion to things we find distasteful, whether it's a child facing yucky vegetables or an adult facing a difficult conversation.

Furthermore, most physicians have an aversion to problems they cannot solve and conditions they cannot control.

Competition for attention. In our crazy-busy world, it's more difficult than ever to grab someone's attention. Customized messages that solve an immediate problem are most likely to get through; other messages get trapped in the spam attention filters.

Medical beliefs. Patients and referring physicians hold beliefs about the value you offer, the efficacy of your recommendations and the way in which patients benefit from your care. Whether or not this belief reflects reality, imagine every person you meet is wearing the t-shirt I saw on a toddler once: "For argument's sake, let's assume I'm right."

Avoid the dreaded ABC's. Have you ever run into someone who tries to control others by accusing, blaming and criticizing? It is not a style that works well. Focus on observed behaviors removed from judgment for the best results.

FACTORS THAT PROMOTE YOUR ABILITY TO PERSUADE

Here are some factors that enhance your charisma and your ability to lead.

1. **Tell stories rather than quote facts**

   Let's say you want to persuade a patient to tell more friends about your services. You could say, "Patients under our care experience a 30% reduction in hospital stays."

   Or you could tell the story of a delighted patient.

   Numbers and logic are the language of the thinking brain; stories and pictures are the language of the feeling brain.

   You have a much better chance of persuading with a story.

   Tell more stories in which others are the heroes. In general, story-telling works better than fact-telling. If your stories poke fun at someone, poke fun at yourself.

   Story-telling is a skill that can be improved. Listen to great story-tellers. Attend a storytelling course. Write down stories. Post a bulletin board in the office in which people can share their stories.

2. **Focus on people who "get it" vs people who don't**

   Whether you are hiring staff, building relationships with SENDERS or attracting patients, your time is better invested in connecting with people who "get it" rather than converting people who don't.

   Steve Jobs said that his main and hardest job was recruiting the right team members. The same hold true for you. You are creating a team of patients, employees, medical specialists, consultants and vendors to support change.

Can You Fire Patients?

You may end a relationship with a patient for many reasons:

- The patient is uncooperative

- The patient is abusive to staff
- The patient is disruptive to the office
- The patient does not keep appointments or pay medical bills
- The patient requires services you do not offer

You may not:

- Discriminate
- Refuse to treat a patient on the basis of their HIV status
- Abandon a patient in the midst of a medical crisis
- Ask your staff to terminate the relationship
- Withhold medical records

Here is the process to terminate a relationship with a patient in a way that upholds professional ethics and offers protection from untoward legal consequences.

Put the patient on written notice that they need to find another healthcare provider. Send this letter by certified mail, and request a return receipt. Place copies of all documents in the patient's chart.

You are not required to offer a reason for termination; however, the absence of an explanation can lead to questions or phone calls. You can frame the conversation in terms of the best interests of the patient. Try, "Despite our best efforts, we are not seeing a clinical improvement. I believe you would be best served by seeking your care from a different physician. I am terminating our relationship effective thirty days from the date of this letter."

Offer to provide medical records to your patient's new healthcare provider. Offer a plan for interim care.

You may terminate the relationship immediately if the patient initially terminated the relationship or they present a threat to you or your staff.

What is the best way to manage this situation? Prevent it! Decide what kind of patient you will not accept into your practice. A psychiatrist's business card says "No Borderlines" after being stalked by a dysfunctional patient with borderline personality disorder.

1. Understand what's important to others.

Again, the best way to get what you want is to help other people get what they want. In general, here's what people want:

- They want to know that you care about them.

- They want to be appreciated.

- They want to be heard.

- They want simplicity.

- They want to be missed.

- They want to know they are not alone.

- They want to be part of something bigger than themselves.

2. Always add value

With each contact that you make, you have a chance to improve the conditions of others in big and small ways. Decide that every person you meet will be just a little better off because they crossed your path. It does not take a lot. Offer a smile or a hand with a door.

3. Help others become more effective leaders

Nordstrom's empowers its sales force to do the right thing. Do you give your staff the autonomy to do the right things for patients and SENDERS? Can you empower family caregivers to assume family leadership? Can you help patients with self-leadership?

4. Understand environmental cues

Create environments that support behavioral changes. If you are serious about eating healthily, it's wise to remove the food you want to avoid and stock up on nutritious food. People who go through drug or alcohol rehab are encouraged to move and change friends. Why? The environment offers cues that support the old bad habits - and not the new good ones.

HOW TO INSPIRE PATIENTS TO FOLLOW-THROUGH

You have the power to do things to and for patients to facilitate a medical transformation. However, the choices patients make when they leave your clinic or the hospital influence the medical outcomes in a profound way.

Some patients have answered their health wake-up calls with transformative lifestyle changes; others do not.

How do you respond when patients politely ignore your doctors' orders?

First, understand that this is more about your patients than it is about you. You may be asking them to change deeply embedded habits.

Second, consider the most effective way to support behavioral change. Vicki was part of a national panel to discuss just this topic. The question was, "What works better: the carrot or the stick?"

She proposed a third option - take a CAB to change: compassion, alternatives and a buddy.

1. **Listen with compassion**. There's a reason that people do the things they do, even if it does not make immediate sense. Be a sleuth and look for the reason.

   Let's say you have a patient who needs to stop smoking. The truth is that smoking is a highly effective stress management tool. Smokers generally leave the environment that creates the stress. They have something to do with their hands and their mouth. They socialize, take deep breaths and induce a relaxing neuro-chemical change. No wonder it's so hard to give up smoking; it works. Well, it works with a price tag that's simply too high.

2. **Find alternatives.** Next, ask your patient, "How can we help you enjoy the same benefits without smoking?" What is the alternative way for a hopeful ex-smoker to leave a stressful environment, have something to do with their mouth and hands, get a social connection, take a deep breath and induce a neurochemical change? It means replacing a habit that impairs health with different habits that serve health - leaving the desk every two hours for a ten-minute walk, or putting on headphones and taking deep breaths or carrying worry beads.

3. **Recruit a buddy.** It's easier to do something if someone holds you accountable. Ask your patient to choose an accountability

buddy. Ask them to make commitments, put them in writing and stand accountable for their actions.

Recognize that many unhealthy habits like smoking, eating donuts or drinking alcohol are attempts at self-medication. Perhaps increasing numbers of people medicate the pain of loneliness. Paradoxically our technology that allows us to connect so effortlessly has left us lacking in meaningful human connections. Maybe that's one reason the buddy system is so important. It's a way of connecting.

Understand why otherwise smart patients make not-so-smart medical choices.

Here are five reasons why even smart patients - including physicians seeking medical care - make not-so-smart choices.

1. **Bad habits.** Why is your patient eating fast food three months after his heart attack? After all, his big wake-up call demonstrated the consequences of burgers and fries. He simply has not freed himself from his lifelong eating habits. Yet.

2. **Blind spots.** We all have them. Your patients simply may not see their growing isolation or the gradual accumulation of pounds. Anais Nin says, "We don't see things as they are; we see things as we are."

3. **Pain and medication.** Your patients' thinking may be clouded by pain, their underlying medical condition or medication. You are at your best in the office; patients are generally at their worst.

4. **Trauma.** Childhood medical traumas can impact individuals for life. A child who was laughed at or shamed when he cried during vaccinations may have a life-long aversion to needles.

5. **Priorities.** Your patients' desire to be seen as a "good patient" may be more important than telling the truth about why they stopped taking their medication. The longing to maintain dignity and be seen as someone who has something to offer can lead to not-so-smart choices.

SUMMARY

- Leaders are change agents.

- Your power to persuade is a skill that you can improve.

- Take a CAB to change: compassion, alternatives and an accountability buddy.

ACTION STEPS:

✓ Define the outcome you are trying to achieve.

✓ Explore your current persuasion tactics.

✓ Invest to become more persuasive.

10

GROOM SELF-LEADERS

Some leaders are born; others are groomed.

THE SEVEN HABITS OF EFFECTIVE HEALERS AND LEADERS

1. **Set the emotional thermostat.**

   As a medical student Vicki was taught that the very first thing doctors do at a cardiac arrest is take their own pulse.

   Moods are catchy. If you're with someone who's scared or anxious you may feel it. It's because our brains are wired with mirror neurons.

   The emotional temperature is important for this reason: emotion drives motion. You have a much better chance of engaging the thinking brain when the emotional climate is set in the range of calm, love and joy.

   Keep the calm rather than catch the chaos.

2. **Let them take center stage.**

   Imagine that any encounter occurs in a theater stage. There is one seat in center stage and plenty of room in the audience. You decide whom you put in center stage - yourself or your conversation partner.

   Put your conversation partner in center stage. As you begin the medical encounter, ask patients, "What are your goals for today's appointment?" If you are speaking with an executive director about a presentation, ask, "How can I help you deliver the most value to your members?"

3. **Shield them from the details.**

   Information is powerful medicine. Make sure that you are administering the right dose.

   Make things simple and clear for patients. Summarize key ideas on one page. Make a drawing. If they ask for details, make them available.

4. **Access your wisdom.**

   You may have treated military people with post-traumatic stress disorder (PTSD). A truck backfires, and it's like they're back in Iraq. Their brains do not understand that the past is over, and that they are safe.

   At any point, your patients may be responding to a traumatic medical situation in the past. Vicki remembers getting her tonsils out as a child. She was left alone in the OR hall most likely just for a few seconds; it felt like an eternity. She was always careful to make sure that her patients never felt alone in scary circumstances.

   Your clients may trip over a trigger that brings them back to a childhood trauma. The smell in a doctor's office may trigger a trauma from your own childhood.

   You can tell this is happening when people just don't act like themselves. Their child-like response is way out of proportion to the event. In fact, they're running the "brain software" that was running at the time of the trauma.

   When you see this happening with a client, gently ask about their childhood medical experiences.

5. **Master the fine art of verbal persuasion.**

   Sometimes it feels more like hostage negotiation.

   Deep listening is the skill that will make you a more persuasive leader.

6. **Know where you're going.**

   Have you ever played Chinese Checkers, and gotten so invigorated in making jumps that you forgot where you were headed to win?

   Help your patients get to their finish line. Activity does not always translate to results. Measure their progress. Show them the transformation. "When you came in the first visit you could not walk up a flight of stairs. Now you're getting ready for a half marathon. Good work."

   Measure your own progress, too. You have a vision of where you want to take your practice. Keep that vision handy. Stephen Covey says that high performers create twice - once in their heads and then again in the outer world.

   Make sure that your activities are taking you in the right direction.

7. **Play it safe; know your limits.**

   Where are some tasks better performed by others? This gives you the freedom to do what you do best. Effective leaders know when to say no.

HOW TO SAY NO - NICELY

Imagine reaching for your cell phone to respond to an emergency. You begin the call and hear the beep that tells you the batteries are low. You're irritated; you lent your phone to a family member, and now when you really need it you can't use it.

What do you say when someone asks for your time or your energy or your attention? The same way you'd respond to a request to borrow your cell phone! Be smart about when and with whom you share.

Here are some tips that will help you say no - nicely.

Remember that "No" is not a four-letter word. The same people who may have heard you utter the seven words George Carlin couldn't say on TV, may rarely hear you say, "No." If you feel like an evil person when you say "no," you're not alone.

Furthermore, while "No" is a complete sentence, you can smoothen the sharp edges by making a "no sandwich."

The "meat" of the message is "I would love to help, but not this time." It's delivered between slices of caring and compassion.

First, communicate that you "get" the other person. Let them know that you have heard them and see the importance of their request. Recognize their pain. "I completely understand why it's so important to get to the meeting. People are counting on you!"

Then deliver "No" seasoned with your desire to help. "I wish I could help. It's just not in the stars today." No need to elaborate. The person who asked does not need to know that you're planning to take a nap or get your long-neglected hair styled.

If you feel guilty about taking care of yourself when someone has a more urgent need, think of plugging your cell phone into the charger. A powerless phone does no one any good.

End with a statement of your support and confidence in their ability to work it out. "I know how resourceful you are. I'm sure you'll find a way to make this happen."

If this is new for you, please know that saying no will feel uncomfortable. That's okay. Just remember you are making sure that you will be there to say yes when it's really important.

Learning how to graciously decline a request helps you stay in the long caregiving marathon. On the flip side, failure to say "no" is the fast track to burn-out.

SUMMARY

- You benefit when you groom your staff and patients to assume leadership.

- The seven habits of effective healers and leaders are key to motivating your staff

ACTION STEPS:

- ✓ Study the seven habits of effective healers and leaders
- ✓ Learn to say "no" effectively

PUTTING IT ALL TOGETHER

You now have a process to transform your practice from where you are now to where you would like it to be. The ideas in this book are like a practice-building History & Physical - a process to facilitate the transformation. This is a system that works.

Do you remember the first few patients you evaluated as a medical student? Vicki spent about 10 hours conducting and writing up her first H&P. To become the skilled physician you are now, you learned a choreographed process for evaluating patients, developed new skills and honed your judgment.

The same holds true with each step in the reinvented medical practice. Some steps will be easier to implement than others.

Elevating the patient experience is your key to success. You can no longer build a thriving practice by simply giving patients what they need; the successful physician will understand what patients and referring physicians truly want and why they want it.

Through this process you will gain clarity about the experience you want to deliver, and empower your staff members to deliver this experience.

You can achieve the personal, professional and financial goals that attracted you to a career in medicine.

We believe that the golden days of medicine are not over; they are just beginning. If we have done our job, you'll see the professional and financial opportunities before you.

Thank you for investing your time into exploring how you can thrive in the Post-Obamacare Era. We believe that you can get back to the dream that attracted you to a career in medicine. We hope that you have found value in the proven strategies and tactics you've learned.

Learning new ideas is an important first step in practice transformation; however, execution leads to change.

Would you like help with implementation? We would be happy to help you with the next steps.

Your very first step is taking control of your cash-flow. Contact a Certified Medical Revenue Manager to assist you in taking control of your cash-flow and plugging the leaks.

APPENDIX A
NEW SELF TALK FOR PHYSICIANS

WARNING: Don't let the simplicity of these words fool you. Self-talk has science behind it (see Patrick's book How to Reprogram Yourself for Success*)! Repeating these words on a daily basis for 30 days can change your life … and the lives of those around you. Change begins inside.*

The way I talk to myself about my practice is extremely important.

Today, I will change the way I think about myself as a doctor and I will begin to think of myself as a successful business owner as well as a caring physician.

I choose to purposely and actively input good thoughts about practicing medicine and I will verbalize them in my mind constantly throughout the day.

I have a positive mental attitude about everything that happens to me and every person that I come in contact with in my practice. I like serving my patients and I find some positive trait in everyone I meet.

Today is going to be one of the most productive, fulfilling experiences of my career. I am going to make the most of every situation, no matter how challenging it might be. Challenges only force me to grow and expand my patience, compassion and love for my patients and my staff.

I know that greatness in medicine begins in the minds of those whose thoughts are positive and self-assured. I know that what I believe about myself is what I will become -- so I believe in the best for myself.

My mind is constantly in tune with the good and the positive. It is bright, cheerful, enthusiastic, and full of good, positive thoughts and ideas about how to make my practice even more successful today and every day.

I am a great physician and what I say and do shows that to others. I am alive and focused. I am mentally alert and wide awake. I feel great and I change the channel when I hear negative comments around me or about me, from patients or from my staff.

I know that I can erase the old programming that has held me back and replace it with new programming that tells my brain what it needs to hear all day long about building a successful medical practice.

My mind is orderly and well-organized. I like to learn about the latest advances in medicine and how to make my practice even more profitable. I consciously choose what I think and I always choose those thoughts which are the most beneficial for me.

I dwell on the future of my practice rather than the past. I put the best connotation on everything and every person I encounter. I expect things to work out successfully and right, and they do!

I am practical and realistic, and I keep my feet on solid ground. But I also give myself the freedom to live up to my fullest expectations as a practicing physician.

My mind dwells only on those thoughts which create more harmony, balance, and well-being within me and in the world around me.

As a physician and a business owner, I automatically, and always, think in a decisive and determined way. When I set my mind to accomplish something, nothing stands in my way.

I am full of resolution and the absolute assurance of the best possible outcome in everything that I do.

I have a good strong winning attitude about myself and about everything I do to build a healthy medical practice.

I choose to look at the world around me in the bright, healthy light of optimism and self-assurance. I know that I have a choice, each day, in my attitude towards my patients and my staff and the things that happen to me each day. I purposely choose to have a cheerful, fun-loving attitude towards everything and everyone I come in contact with. This keeps me positive, upbeat and happy throughout the day.

I know that what I say to myself throughout the day is very important, and I always say things that are positive and encouraging to myself and to others.

If I have ever had any doubts about myself as a successful owner of a medical practice, today is a good day to put them aside, and I'm doing just that by repeating these positive, self-edifying words.

It's a good day to throw out any disbelief that ever held me back and I am cleaning out the old garbage and replacing it with new words and thoughts right now.

I know that I am headed in the right winning direction in my practice, and I look forward and never look back. I have the ability to focus on one thing at a time, so I concentrate my attention on the job at hand and I get it done!

I control the thoughts I choose. No thought, at any time, can dwell in my mind without my approval or permission. I never worry about anything. I focus on the solution to every problem and challenge that comes my way.

All I need to do, on a regular basis, is to listen to and repeat in my mind these winning words that can change the way I think about myself, and I can be the successful physician I deserve to be, starting this very day.

Right now, even while I am telling myself these truths about me, I know that I can succeed and I am succeeding at building a thriving medical practice. At this moment, if I think of any challenge in front of me, I know that I will become even more a winner because of it.

I keep my chin up, my head held high. I look, act, sound, think, and feel like the winner I am! Anytime a problem starts to get me down, I get myself right back up! I tackle problems and I solve them. When frustration or defeat threatens me, I just become that much stronger, more positive, better organized, and more determined than ever!

Right now, today, this very moment, I am capable of giving myself the gift of absolute self-assurance, self-belief, and powerful non-stop confidence in myself. By just saying these words to myself I create these positive changes in myself.

No matter what it is that requires the very best of me, I can do it and I know I can.

I know it's all up to me. One hundred percent and every bit of it. All of it is in how I look at it and what I do about it! That's what winning is. That's why I am a winner. That's because positive self-talk really does change the way I think about myself and my practice.

I know happiness comes from inside, so I think and say things that keep me focused on the happiness of the moment – just the thrill of being alive, and knowing that my future is bright.

I set my sights. I keep my balance. I don't hesitate. I don't hold back! I know that the building a successful practice is full of opportunities.

Just look at what joy and hope I can bring to others, today! I am an incredible doctor . . . and today is a great day to show it to my patients and to my staff!

I can do anything I believe I can do! I've got lots of confidence in my abilities as a physician and as a business owner, and every day I get more of it.

I set goals and I reach them. I know what I want out of my medical practice. I go after it and I get what I want. I never hurt others in my pursuit of my goals. I encourage my patients by what I do and say to achieve their best health.

Every word I say to myself about myself is exactly how I am, right now. I can improve in lots of different areas, but I like who I am right now.

I am exactly who I think I am – therefore, I will never stop thinking good thoughts about me.

Nothing seems to stop me. I have a lot of determination. I turn problems into advantages. I find possibilities in things that other people would never think of as having potential.

I have a lot of energy. I am very alive! I enjoy life and I can tell it and so can others. I keep myself up, looking ahead, and liking it.

I know that I can accomplish anything I choose, and I refuse to let anything negative hold me back or stand in my way.

I am not afraid of anything or anyone. I have strength, power, conviction, and confidence! I like challenges and I meet them head on, face to face -- today especially!

I am on top of the world and I'm going for it. I have a clear picture in my mind of what I want in my medical practice. I can see it in front of me. I know what I want and I go for it.

I really am very special. I like who I am and I feel good about myself. Others see me as a loving, caring person, and I am. I let my patients know that I care for them in all that I say and do when I'm with them.

I wanted to be a physician and run a successful and profitable medical practice - and now I know I can. Everything I do is designed specifically to build a practice that is a model in my community.

I am positive. I am confident. I radiate good things. My staff can see how positive I am by what I say and how I react to little things all day long.

I am full of life. I like life and I'm glad to be alive. I am a very special person, living at a very special time. The advances in medicine keep me motivated and anxious to learn how to be a better physician every day.

Although at times challenges or difficulties may arise, I conquer them with my positive constructive approach and calmness.

I am intelligent. My mind is quick and alert and clever and fun. I think good thoughts, and my mind makes things work right for me.

I have a lot of energy and enthusiasm and vitality. I am exciting and I really enjoy being me.

I like to be around other people and other people like to be around me. People like to hear what I have to say and know what I have to think.

I smile a lot. I am happy on the inside and I am happy on the outside. I have a great sense of humor and my staff and my patients love to be near me.

I am interested in many things. I appreciate all the blessings I have, and the things that I learn, and all the things I will learn today and tomorrow and every day.

I am warm, sincere, honest, and genuine. I am all of these things and more. And all of these things are me. I like who I am, and I'm glad to be me!

I know that improving my thoughts is the best way to improve my life and my practice. What I think about, I become.

APPENDIX B
RESOURCES

BOOKS

How to Reprogram Yourself for Success, Patrick Phillips

The E-Myth Revisited, Michael Gerber

E-Myth Mastery: The Seven Essential Disciplines for Building a World Class Company, Michael Gerber

Made to Stick: Why Some Ideas Survive and Others Die, Chip Heath, Dan Heath

Good to Great: Why Some Companies Make the Leap... and Others Don't, Jim Collins

The 4-Hour Workweek: Escape 9-5, Live Anywhere, and Join the New Rich, Timothy Ferriss

The New Rules of Marketing and PR: How to Use Social Media, Blogs, News Releases, Online Video, and Viral Marketing to Reach Buyers Directly, David Meerman Scott

Finding Your Own North Star: Claiming the Life You Were Meant to Live, Martha Beck

Tribes: We Need You to Lead Us, Seth Godin

A Whole New Mind: Why Right-Brainers Will Rule the Future, Daniel H. Pink

Entrepreneur's Notebook: Practical Advice for Starting a New Business Venture, Steven K. Gold

The Purple Cow, Seth Godin

Blue Ocean Strategy, Expanded Edition: How to Create Uncontested Market Space and Make the Competition Irrelevant, W. Chan Kim and Renée Mauborgne

Better: A Surgeon's Notes on Performance, Atul Gawande

The Checklist Manifesto: How to Get Things Right, Atul Gawande

Complications: A Surgeon's Notes on an Imperfect Science, Atul Gawande

Twitter Power 2.0: How to Dominate Your Market One Tweet at a Time, Joel Comm

The Long Tail: Why the Future of Business is Selling Less of More, Chris Anderson

The Power of Why: Breaking Out in a Competitive Marketplace, C. Richard Weylman

The Five Love Languages: The Secret to Love that Lasts, Gary D Chapman

The Meaning of Money: Creating Not Just Wealth on Your Balance Sheet But Significance in Your Life, Rao Garuda

LINKS

Medical Revenue Management Association of America – mrmaa.org

Medical Bridges – medicalbridges.com

Thriving Doctors Bootcamp – thrivingdoctors.com

Examples of great storytellers – ted.org

Great source for contractors – fiverr.com

NEWSLETTERS

Revenue Cycle Intelligence – revenuecycleintelligence.com

Physician's Practice - physicianspractice.com/publication

Medical Economics – medicaleconomics.modernmedicine.com

Physician's Money Digest - hcplive.com/physicians-money-digest

INDEX